HOW TO STAY OUT OF THE HOSPITAL

HOW TO STAY OUT OF THE HOSPITAL

A Practical Guide to Healthy Options and Alternatives

by Lila L. Anastas, R.N.

Rodale Press   Emmaus, Pennsylvania

Printed in the United States of America on recycled paper, containing a high percentage of de-inked fiber.

Book design by Darla Hoffman

Library of Congress Cataloging in Publication Data

Anastas, Lila.
    How to stay out of the hospital.

    Includes index.
    1. Medical care. 2. Hospital care. 3. Medical
errors. 4. Consumer education. I. Title.
[DNLM: 1. Attitude to Health—popular works.
2. Hospitalization—popular works. 3. Professional-
Patient Relations—popular works. WX 158.5 A534h]
RA413.A616   1986   613   85–30064

ISBN 0-87857-609-6   hardcover
ISBN 0-87857-610-X   paperback

2 4 6 8 10 9 7 5 3 1   hardcover
2 4 6 8 10 9 7 5 3 1   paperback

NOTICE

This book is intended as a reference volume only, not as a medical manual or guide to self-treatment. If you suspect that you have a medical problem, we urge you to seek competent medical help. The information here is intended to help you make informed decisions about your health.

To my father,
Granville W. Larimore, MD,
for his constant encouragement
in my career
and in my personal life

CONTENTS

PREFACE

I'm one of 1.4 million people in this country who can use the title Registered Nurse after his or her name. I'm proud of that fact.

In the almost 25 years that I've been a member of the nursing profession, there have been many changes in how health care is given in this country. The technological advances that have occurred are staggering. Critical care units, with their complex lifesaving equipment, could only be imagined 25 years ago. The use of computers for diagnosis and the success of organ transplants and open heart surgery—these are all new phenomena that have given hope to millions of people.

This is the age of specialization and high technology. But it's also the age of chaotic, fragmented, impersonalized, and very expensive health care. To borrow from Dickens, it is the best of times and the worst of times.

Today, more than ever, it is essential that you take a more active role in your health care. This begins with keeping fit, extends to preventing illness, and ends in selecting the right health care provider among the many alternatives that are now available. In some cases it means making a decision as to whether to enter a hospital.

One of my duties as a nurse is to act as a patient advocate—to help sort out the conflicting advice in the best interests of the patient. What that often boils down to is helping a patient decide whether the benefits of taking a certain action will outweigh the risks involved.

You may, for example, be faced with the question of elective surgery. Should you have your uterus or gallbladder or tonsils removed if a surgeon recommends it? Of course, you say, the doctor knows best. But in a special report by the House Interstate and Foreign Commerce Committee titled "The Cost and Quality of Health Care: Unnecessary Surgery," it was found that of the 14 million *elective* operations performed each year, 17 percent, or 2.4 million, are unnecessary. These unnecessary operations cost $4 billion and result in 12,000 patient deaths every year.

A 1976 incident in Southern California provided a "natural experiment" that lends even more support to the harmful effects of elective surgery. From January 1 to February 4, 1976, a substantial number of doctors in Los Angeles County withheld their services for mostly nonemergency surgery (patients continued to receive emergency medical and surgical care). This "doctor strike" was a reaction to escalating premiums for malpractice insurance. Daily newspaper accounts suggested "harmful effects" for patients in the Los Angeles area. But, according to a study by Roemer and Schwartz presented at the 1978 American Public Health Association meeting, the only harmful effects of the medical slowdown appeared to be on the doctors' and hospitals' incomes.

Effects on potential patients were very beneficial. The withholding of nonemergency surgery was associated with a significant reduction in the county's overall death rate, compared with each of the previous five years. For the first week that normal surgical practice was resumed, there was a substantial jump in the death rate. These findings, and others like them, have led many to believe that elective surgical procedures can do more harm than good.

Do you still want to have elective surgery? Have you sought a second opinion? Have the risks of surgery been pointed out to you? Do you know what will happen if you don't have the surgery? Is there a more conservative course of treatment that can be tried first? As an informed health consumer, these are some of the questions you should ask your surgeon. And the doctor's answers—along with other sources and your own common sense—should help you to make the right decision *for you*.

It is not my purpose in writing this book to scare anyone. As a health consumer myself, I'm very upset when I read a newspaper account of still another medical horror story. But, unfortunately, these are as much a part of reality as the medical miracles that occur every day. I will include both kinds of anecdotes in this book.

Many generous people willingly gave their time and shared their thoughts and experiences with me. In order to protect the privacy of patients, all names have been changed in the anecdotal or case history sections. The names of most health care workers also have been changed except for those persons who are referred to in a specific work setting.

This book contains valuable information on the new alternatives to hospitalization. It also explains how you can receive the best care if you or a family member are hospitalized because of an accident or serious illness.

It is my hope that, after reading this book, you will be able to make a more informed choice about entering a hospital. The day is past when you can blindly put your total faith and trust in the health care system. There are too many variables, too many problems, and most important, too much at stake.

Your health care is serious business. It's a matter of life and death.

Chapter 1

CAUTION: HOSPITALS CAN BE HAZARDOUS TO YOUR HEALTH

"Oh my God," said the surgeon as bright red blood spurted all over the operative field.

"I think I got the artery!"

In the process of removing a stone from the patient's ureter, the surgeon had inadvertently cut into the renal artery. After borrowing a pair of glasses from a nurse (he had left his own at home but operated anyway), the surgeon spent 10 to 15 minutes mopping and floundering before he clamped off the artery and repaired the damage. Although this happened several years ago, the explanation that the surgeon gave to the patient's husband could be the same today as it was then. "The surgery was very difficult, but I think we saved your wife."

The truth of the matter was that, even though the woman was lucky to have survived the surgery, as a result of it she never had proper circulation to her kidney and suffered poor health for the rest of her life.

In a busy Detroit hospital two patients named Johnson were scheduled for surgery on the same day. M. Johnson was to have a hernia repair, while S. Johnson's operation was to be for hemorrhoids. The first Johnson was inadvertently prepared for hemorrhoid surgery (he also had hemorrhoids). Halfway through surgery the error was recognized, and after the procedure was finished, the patient was turned over and redraped, and the hernia repair was done. I leave it to the reader's imagination as to how the surgeon explained his way out of this mix-up and the resultant stormy convalescence.

Leaving sponges behind, operating on the wrong leg. These are standard hospital "jokes," but they're far from funny for the patients involved. The impersonal, chaotic atmosphere of every modern hospital lends itself to errors being made. And physicians are not the only ones who make them.

At one busy Midwestern hospital, an overburdened night nurse was passing the early morning medications. She had two injections to administer—insulin to a diabetic and vitamin B_{12} to an anemic patient. Both women were elderly and had been in the hospital for some time. Both had lost or removed their ID bracelets and both wandered the halls in the early morning hours disoriented and confused. The nurse inadvertently administered the wrong medications—the diabetic woman received the B_{12} and the patient with anemia got the insulin. The first was almost unconscious and the second very ill before the error was noted by the day shift and proper remedial action taken. An incident report was written up by the nurse, but the families were never told about the mix-up.

In still another hospital the night nurse inadvertently forgot to pull up the siderails on a patient's high bed. Sleeping fitfully because of medication, the patient rolled out of bed, fell on the floor, and fractured his skull.

I have specifically used the word "inadvertently" in all these real situations because in every case the mistakes were not intentional. But they happened.

In recent years there has been increasing publicity about the mistakes that physicians and other health team members make. Even more upsetting to patients have been the conspiracy of silence and the cover-ups that follow such mistakes.

Patients now take out their anger by suing the physician, the nurse, the hospital, the pharmaceutical or medical equipment company. The list is endless. I doubt that anyone, except malpractice lawyers and insurance companies, benefits from this approach.

Statistically, it's only a small minority of hospital patients who suffer such serious mishaps as the ones just described. But mistakes are an all-too-frequent problem in today's health institutions, so many of which are understaffed and disorganized. And if a mistake happens to you, the statistics are 100 percent.

Here's the hospital story—horror story, really—of a man who was the victim of multiple mistakes.

ONE PATIENT'S BIZARRE STORY

Joe and Diana Merrick, who are in their late 30s, have two young children and live in Southern California. Joe has been healthy all his life, has watched his diet, and has exercised regularly.

Last Memorial Day, Joe and Diana spent the weekend doing odd jobs around their house. The work hadn't been strenuous, but Tuesday morning, when it was time to go to work, Joe's lower back hurt so badly that he could hardly get out of bed. Thinking it was a result of overdoing, he decided the pain would go away in a few days. But when a week went by and he was still no better, he saw his family physician, who diagnosed the problem as a muscle strain and prescribed muscle relaxants (cost of the visit: $40). After another week there was still no relief, so Joe made an appointment to see a chiropractor. The chiropractor took x-rays and felt he could help Joe with manipulative treatments. Twice a week for three weeks, Joe visited the chiropractor. At several sessions traction was used. But nothing helped (cost: $268). So, Joe went to Dr. Goodman, an orthopedist who told him right off that he never should have gone to the chiropractor. Dr. Goodman suspected a slipped disk and took another set of spinal x-rays ($100). Although the x-rays weren't conclusive, Dr. Goodman felt that his diagnosis was correct and sent Joe to a physical therapist. Three times a week Joe received treatments from the therapist. For two weeks it was exercises and ultrasound, then traction was begun. The pain was excruciating.

After he returned home from one session, Diana found Joe on the floor experiencing chest pains and difficulty breathing. For three days the Merricks tried to contact Dr. Goodman, but he was out of town and their messages never got past the answering service. So Joe went back to the physical therapist, who explained that it wasn't uncommon to have chest pains while undergoing traction. As Joe remembers it, the therapist gave him this strange explanation: "When you stand up fast, the spinal fluid shoots up and brings on a sensation like chest pain." Joe assumed the therapist knew what he was talking about, so he continued for several more treatments (a total of four weeks of physical therapy at $560).

But the back pains had shifted higher up Joe's spine and the chest pains continued. The Merricks called Dr. Goodman's office, but once again he was out of town. This time, however, the orthopedist on call—Dr. Simmons—saw Joe and was concerned enough about the chest pains to admit him to the local hospital. Joe was seen by a cardiologist, who saw no indication of a heart attack. While Joe was in the hospital, Dr. Simmons ordered another set of spinal x-rays, this time of the upper vertebrae. The x-rays suggested a fracture, and a bone scan was done to confirm the diagnosis. After two days and one night in the hospital (cost: $783), Joe was released with a diagnosis of a fractured vertebra. The doctors felt that the chiropractor was probably responsible for the fracture.

Joe remembers one aspect of this hospitalization very vividly: "When I was admitted, I was having chest pains and difficulty breathing. I'm a nonsmoker and requested either a private room or a room with another nonsmoker. Instead, they assigned me to a five-bed ward with four chain smokers in the other beds. Believe me, I couldn't wait to get out of there!"

For one week after his trip to the hospital Joe stayed home— lying flat in bed and taking medication for pain. In the meantime Dr. Goodman had returned to town and didn't like Dr. Simmons' diagnosis of a fractured vertebra. He saw Joe in his office and ran a number of tests ($150). The urine test showed an infection, so Joe was referred to a urologist. After another urine test, no infection was found ($118).

Dr. Goodman still maintained that Joe had a slipped disk, and wanted to do a CAT—computerized axial tomography—scan (a special x-ray) to diagnose the problem. By this time Joe was becoming disenchanted with Dr. Goodman and wanted to be under Dr. Simmons' care. Joe called Dr. Simmons' office but was told that this was a very difficult situation, and to maintain harmony between the two physicians, it would be best for Joe to stay with Dr. Goodman. So Joe stuck with Dr. Goodman and had the CAT scan done as an outpatient ($400). It didn't show a slipped disk, so Dr. Goodman confessed that he really didn't know what the problem was and referred Joe to Dr. Steiger, an orthopedist who specialized in spinal problems.

Dr. Steiger examined his new patient and noticed that there was a sore on Joe's thumb. The sore, oddly enough, had begun before

Memorial Day, but none of the other doctors had felt it was significant. The sore led Dr. Steiger to suspect that Joe had an unusual infectious condition that was a result of a recurring childhood back injury. But the test for this condition was done and results were negative. Dr. Steiger ordered a tomograph and a gallium scan ($587), which showed activity in the vertebral space. (The CAT scan, tomograph, and gallium scan were all used to help diagnose Joe's problem. The CAT scan combines x-ray equipment, which directs beams into the body from nearly 300 different angles, with a computer, which analyzes the information and visually reconstructs cross sections of the inside of the body. Tomography records a detailed description of what a thin slice of the patient looks like. Many tomograph slices make up a CAT scan. A gallium scan uses radioactive contrast material that will concentrate in certain organs. If there is an infection or abscess, it should show up as a black mass. These tests are often used together to check one result against another. They may also be repeated to follow the course of a patient's condition.)

The new diagnosis was an infection in the disk space. So, infection specialists (five in the group) were called in ($260) and they decided to admit Joe once again to the hospital.

Under general anesthesia, Dr. Steiger did microscopic surgery on Joe's spine. First the surgeon withdrew some spinal fluid and took tissue samples from the disk. At the same time, they opened up the infected thumb and scraped the bone to get a tissue sample. These samples—from the back and the thumb—were sent to the laboratory to determine the infectious organisms. In spite of the fact that nothing showed up in the cultures, antibiotic therapy was begun. Amoxicillin was administered intravenously for six weeks, and the thumb was soaked in Betadine four times a day for several weeks.

These procedures were not without difficulty. Following the operation, Joe's blood pressure dropped significantly and was a cause of much concern. At one point during the intravenous therapy, Joe's IV infiltrated and the pain, which spread up to his shoulder, lasted for several days. The Amoxicillin upset his stomach, with the result that he ate very little and lost weight.

For some reason that escapes the Merricks, a dermatologist was called in to examine Joe's thumb. During the course of his examination he noted a flaking of the skin on Joe's head and suspected psoriasis. He prescribed a steroid cream. When the infection specialists found out, they would not allow him to use it.

Meanwhile, the infection team was leaning toward a diagnosis of osteomyelitis (bone infection) and performed a second operation on Joe's thumb (this time under local anesthesia). The surgeons removed part of the bone, with the result that the thumb no longer functions as well as it did. Although the doctors felt that the thumb was badly infected, tests once again showed no infection. Continual tests of the blood sedimentation rate showed an elevation at the time of admission, a gradual decline, and then a leveling off (measurement of the sedimentation rate is a nonspecific screening test; the rate may be elevated in infection, inflammatory disease, and other conditions). Meanwhile, another tomograph and gallium scan were ordered for Joe's back, but the results showed there was no change from the previous test.

What was wrong with both Joe's back *and* thumb still eluded the doctors but they didn't stop looking for *the* diagnosis. They called in two new specialists. The new orthopedist wasn't sure what the problem was but recommended exploratory spinal surgery, although this would lay Joe up for months (Dr. Steiger vetoed the idea). The new infection specialist thought Joe might be suffering from a collagen disease. This was an intriguing notion to *all* the doctors. (A collagen disease is any of a number of clinical conditions characterized by widespread alterations of connective tissue, including inflammation and fibrinoid degeneration). A few more tests were done. Could it be undulant fever? Tests said no.

The cost of the second hospital stay, thus far, was $17,000.

With still no definitive diagnosis and with little relief from his back pain, Joe was released from the hospital. He was told to take oral Amoxicillin for one month and gradually return to normal activities (including work).

Following the office visit with Dr. Steiger, Joe had another CAT scan and tomograph at a cost of $715. There was no change from the previous tests.

In a four-month period Joe was seen by at least 14 doctors; had two surgical procedures, three sets of x-rays, one bone scan, three CAT scans, three tomographs, and two gallium scans; and spent 31 days in the hospital. The total cost of his illness (at the time of hospital discharge) was $20,721.

Joe's wife, Diana, tells her side of the story: "I had little faith in most of the doctors. The constantly changing diagnoses and treatment plans were very confusing. And in the hospital we felt we had no choices—everything was out of our hands. The hospital and doctors were definitely in control."

It was only *after* Joe left the hospital that he finally found out what was wrong with him. As a last recourse (and because he was still in pain), Joe was referred to a rheumatologist. At first Joe was reluctant to see this new specialist because he thought it meant steroid therapy. But the new doctor, Dr. Hughes, proceeded slowly. He reviewed all the hospital records and examined his patient carefully. On one visit Joe mentioned to Dr. Hughes that his ears sometimes turned bright red for no particular reason. According to Joe, "That was the clue that Hughes had been looking for. He diagnosed my problem as relapsing polychondritis—a disease that seldom settles in the spine, although mine did. The doctor prescribed the drug Feldene, and shortly after that the disease went into remission. Hughes recently discharged me and I feel great. I've even started running again."

It's been almost a year since Joe's troubles began. In the beginning especially, his family experienced a lot of anxiety and upsetting times. The hospital stay was the most trying time of all.

As Joe Merrick's case points out, once you're in a hospital, it's hard to get out. The doctors' curiosity about his diagnosis became *the* thing, whereas Joe's comfort and well-being were secondary. In all honesty, there was little reason for Joe to stay in the hospital as long as he did (some may question whether he ever needed to be hospitalized). It was convenient for all the doctors to have Joe there—in a bed—where they could check on him while checking other patients, and order another test or procedure. There was a staff of nurses and personnel who could carry out orders and provide coverage for a 24-hour period and there was a consulting staff that was always ready to provide advice and protection. Finally, Joe's insurance company was willing to pay for it all—no questions asked.

If the attending physician and the insurance company could have been persuaded of the benefits, Joe could have stayed right at home. All the tests and minor surgery could have been done on an outpatient basis, and IV therapy could have been carried out at home with nursing assistance. The monetary savings would have been significant. (According to figures cited by the *American Journal of Nursing* in March 1984, the average cost of home IV antibiotic therapy per day is $209, compared with the mean hospital charge of $410 per day. In the average 18.2 days of home IV therapy, the saving per patient would be $3,658.20.)

If Joe had been cared for at home, chances are he would have gotten well faster. He also wouldn't have missed as much work. Being at home would have been easier on his family too. But Joe's physician, whom he trusted, strongly recommended hospitalization. And Joe had the insurance to pick up the tab.

Joe is not too keen on hospitalization now. He knows some of the reasons why other routes should be tried before taking the one to the admitting office. And so should you.

HOSPITAL "CARE" CAN MAKE YOU SICKER

In Joe Merrick's case the drop in blood pressure following surgery, the gastrointestinal upset during antibiotic therapy, and the loss of thumb motion following removal of part of his bone are all examples of iatrogenic illness—illness *caused* by a physician or by medical treatment. It's a problem more common than you might think.

Iatrogenic illness was studied at a Boston teaching hospital, and results were reported in the *New England Journal of Medicine*. Thirty-six percent of the patients at this hospital suffered an iatrogenic illness during their hospital stay. More than 40 percent of these patients had between two and seven adverse reactions to therapy, and 5 percent of the patients actually died as a result. The authors of the study concluded that the risk of an iatrogenic illness among these patients was greater than the risk of heart attack in the general population! This alone is enough to give you second thoughts about voluntarily admitting yourself to the hospital.

Iatrogenic illness can, of course, occur outside the hospital too (like in the doctor's office) but it is less likely to be as serious, because hospital patients are usually sicker to begin with and are usually bedridden. In the hospital, tests are often invasive, surgical procedures are serious, and infections can occur more easily.

Infections You Can Get

In fact, one of the worst problems for all hospitalized patients *is* infection. According to the National Institutes of Health, from 5 to 15 percent of all people who enter a hospital will end up with a nosocomial (hospital-related) infection. This infection will extend their hospital stay an average of seven days. More significantly, at least 15,000 to 20,000 people will die each year because of nosocomial infection. Also, statistics show, you're more likely to pick up one of these infections in a large metropolitan medical center than in a small community hospital.

About 40 percent of all hospital-related infections are those involving the urinary tract. These are usually the result of urinary catheterization (insertion of a tube to drain off urine when a patient is unable to urinate normally). With more careful techniques, however, the incidence of urinary tract infections could be greatly reduced.

One estimate from the Centers for Disease Control is that 5 to 12 percent of all surgical patients develop postoperative wound infections. The incidence, however, can reach 30 percent after certain operations, such as amputation or large-bowel surgery. As in urinary tract infections, the causative organisms are most often gram-negative bacteria, although *Staphylococcus aureus* still plays an important role. Most staphylococcal infections seem to develop from exposure on the recuperating areas after surgery rather than from exposure during the operation. And the longer the preoperative hospital stay, the greater the incidence of infection. The duration of the operation itself can influence the chances of infection. The incidence of wound infection is 5 percent for operations requiring less than 30 minutes, but jumps to 23 percent for operations requiring more than two hours. Infections are also more likely to occur following operations performed between midnight and 8 A.M. Other factors include surgical techniques, types of equipment used, and even punctured surgical gloves.

Nosocomial pneumonias rank third in incidence of hospital-related infections, and the mortality is high. Most affected patients already have a serious underlying disease and many are receiving broad-spectrum antibiotics. These pneumonias are often related to the use of respiratory devices to aid breathing or to administer anesthetics. Such machines are frequently difficult to sterilize effectively.

Still another type of nosocomial infection is bacteremia (the presence of living bacteria in the blood). Usually implicated in this type of infection is intravenous catheterization, or use of IVs. As in urinary catheterization, infection is more likely to occur the longer the catheter remains in place.

Some patients are more likely to develop hospital-related infections than others. Susceptibility is influenced by the nature of the illness or injury, age and general condition of the patient, and type of treatment given. Burn patients, diabetics, the very young, and the old fall into the high-risk group. Even more susceptible to hospital-related infections are those whose immune systems have been altered by drugs or by an underlying disease. Patients undergoing organ transplant operations and cancer patients are particularly prone to infections.

As if hospitalized patients don't have enough trouble with infections already, there's another danger that lurks in the cooling towers, shower heads, and water taps of some hospitals: Legionnaires' disease.

Legionnaires' disease killed 29 people who attended the 1976 American Legion Convention in Philadelphia. Since then, isolated cases of the disease have been reported in various United States hospitals, although the disease generally goes unreported. Many doctors don't think to test for it, diagnosing it simply as pneumonia.

In April 1985, 37 people died of Legionnaires' disease in a new hospital in Stafford, England.

The organism that causes Legionnaires' disease (a bacterium called *Legionella pneumophila*) lives in water and is transmitted by being inhaled. When the air-conditioning cooling towers or water taps are to blame, the water supply must be heavily chlorinated to kill the bacteria.

Researchers at the Centers for Disease Control in Atlanta estimate that Legionnaires' disease strikes 25,000 Americans each year and is fatal in about 15 percent of cases. But these figures are not precise, since it is felt that most cases aren't reported.

The Risks of Surgery

Going to the hospital can be risky business. And surgery is one of the riskiest procedures of all. Approximately 20 to 25 million operations are performed every year in the United States. There is an estimated 1.33 percent mortality involved with these surgeries (in actual numbers, that's at least 300,000 people who lose their lives). But even if the patient survives, the complications of hemorrhage, infection, and damage to major organs can reduce the quality of life for the individual.

One major risk of surgery is anesthesia, the procedures used to put the person to sleep before undergoing the operation. Death or permanent damage can result not from the operation itself, but from the anesthesia. That's why the anesthesiologist is a very important member of the operating team. Considering this, it seems somewhat strange that a patient can go to great lengths to select the "best" surgeon for this job and not give a second thought to the person sending him off to sleep. Yet the anesthesiologist may single-handedly determine the success or failure of an operation.

According to Siegfried J. Kra, MD, in *Examine Your Doctor,* "Ten thousand people die each year from anesthesia and about 2,000 of these did not need surgery in the first place. Death is mainly the result of cardiac arrest and insufficient oxygen reaching the brain and heart. Inadequate deliveries of oxygen to the brain can cause chronic brain damage, coma, dementia, and irreversible damage to body organs. Other complications include eye damage, spinal-cord paralysis with complete paralysis of the body, kidney failure, liver failure, and aspiration into the lungs, resulting in pneumonia and death." That's a lot of risk from one small—albeit important—surgical procedure!

Transfusion Confusion

Untoward reactions can also occur when blood transfusions are given, either in conjunction with surgery or for a medical problem.

In this country 13 million units of blood are collected each year, and 3.5 million persons receive blood or blood products. This number is steadily increasing.

The patient who is severely hemorrhaging absolutely needs blood replacement in order to stay alive. But the hemorrhaging patient is not the only one who receives blood transfusions.

In most hospitals there is a definite protective protocol that is followed when blood is administered. But even with the best precautions, things can go wrong.

Joan Cleveland was in the hospital receiving whole blood for an anemic condition. About five minutes after the blood started flowing through her veins, her head began to ache and she felt a little dizzy. Then she had the sensation that "the inside of my skin was crawling out."

Joan Cleveland was experiencing a mild allergic reaction to the blood transfusion, so her physician discontinued the procedure and instituted other treatment for her anemia. Although allergic reactions can be more serious, they are not the only problem that patients risk. Some other examples:

- *Hemolytic reactions (destruction of blood cells)*—These occur most frequently when a patient is given blood that is incompatible with his system. An Rh-positive patient may, for example, receive Rh-negative blood. Hemolytic reactions usually occur during or immediately following a blood transfusion and start with restlessness and anxiety, complaints of chest pain, tingling sensations, rapid pulse, nausea, vomiting, and shock. Hemolytic reactions can be extremely serious and may lead to death. When a patient is under general anesthesia and is receiving a blood transfusion, most of the symptoms will be masked—this obviously becomes an even more dangerous situation.

- *Circulatory overloading*—This problem is most common in patients with heart disease, and heart failure may be the result.
- *Air embolism*—The transmission of large amounts of air into the vein is potentially dangerous, causing foaming of blood in the heart with consequent inefficiency of pumping. The result: heart failure.
- *Disease transmission*—Most recently, some blood supplies have been contaminated with acquired immune deficiency syndrome (AIDS) virus, and recipients have contracted the disease. In addition, patients may come down with viral hepatitis, bacterial infections, or malaria following a blood transfusion.

One method of avoiding these potential blood transfusion problems is by using autologous transfusions, in which the patients receive their own blood. In a planned surgical procedure, the patient's blood can be drawn some time before surgery, stored, and then given at the time of the operation. But autologous transfusions can be employed only if the patient is in good health. Most often, though, a person receives blood donated from another person. This is in the form of whole blood, which can be stored only for a short period of time and used on an as-needed basis.

Instead of whole blood, a patient may be given plasma (the liquid part of the blood that remains after the cells are removed). However, this is not without risk. A blue-ribbon panel assembled by the National Institutes of Health recently met in Washington and spoke out against the overuse of blood plasma. According to this group, as much as 90 percent of blood plasma use is unwarranted. They suggested doctors turn to alternative substances that offer less risk of transmitting disease. The panel estimated that 3 to 10 percent of patients receiving blood products get hepatitis. There also is a small risk of getting AIDS through transfusions. Of the 6,000 cases of

AIDS reported as of 1984 in the United States, 82 were related to transfusions, the panel said. (A recently developed test for donated blood gives promise of greatly reducing the risk of acquiring AIDS through a blood transfusion.)

The group of experts, led by Dr. James L. Tullis of the Harvard Medical School, said there is little medical evidence to justify the tenfold increase in the use of plasma during the past decade. For example, plasma is used in treating blood volume loss due to injury that could lead to shock. Panel members said salt solutions and other liquids could be used instead to correct decreased fluid volume. The risk of infection increases as a patient gets blood products from multiple donors, and decreasing the use of plasma—which cannot be sterilized—would reduce the sources of possible infection.

Hospitals Can Make You Depressed

Crying. Loss of self-esteem. A sense of helplessness. These are some common symptoms of depression and they occur in approximately one-third of all surgical patients.

Depression, by itself, is a bad enough malady, but coupled with the existing physical problems of the surgical patient it can mean longer time spent in the hospital, more complications, and even increased mortality.

What causes postoperative depression? Some possible causes are surgery that mutilates body parts and causes a change in self-image; pain; and loss of control in the hospital environment. In addition, drugs that are routinely given for surgical procedures, including pain medications and muscle relaxants, can cause depression in some patients. Steroids, antihypertensive drugs, beta blockers, and other heart medications also have been indicted as causes of depression.

Unfortunately, like other emotional issues connected with hospitalization, the depression that follows surgery often goes undetected or is passed off as "nothing to worry about."

OH, THE INDIGNITIES!

Jim McGuire was a successful trial attorney who took pride in handling things "his way." His high-stress job brought on a stomach ulcer, and late one Monday morning he started vomiting blood. Jim called his physician, who told him to report immediately to the local emergency room. From the urgent tone of his doctor's voice, Jim expected that things would move along quickly once he got to the hospital. Not so. First, although his doctor told him that he was to be admitted, the clerk had no record of that fact. After many phone calls, Jim's wife was sent to the admitting office, where she had to complete lengthy paperwork. Meanwhile a nurse took Jim into a curtained-off area and helped him remove his clothes. "No need," said Jim, but the nurse insisted. The "Johnny shirt" had no strings to hold it together, and even though Jim was not a particularly modest person, he felt that he might as well be naked for all the covering the hospital shirt offered. Jim eased onto the hard narrow examining table and waited. The nurse had covered him with a sheet, but he was cold. And he felt very sick.

He lay there thinking the worst. After an hour his doctor arrived, and Jim was transferred to the surgical floor, where people in white coats and uniforms buzzed in and out of his room. A dinner tray was put on his bedside table, then just as quickly was taken out. More blood was drawn, an IV was started, and a tube was passed through his nose into his stomach. More doctors came in to poke and probe.

Jim had eaten nothing since the night before. His head and stomach ached, his mouth was fuzzy, he felt weak as a kitten and terribly alone. Trying to forget his discomfort, he dozed off but was awakened with another needle stick in his arm. "Won't be a minute—doctor needs more blood," mumbled the technician.

Jim lost his temper. "Damn it! I need my blood more than you do! Can't you guys just leave me alone?"

The technician scrambled out the door, and within minutes a nurse—whom Jim had never seen before—marched in and served him a lecture on "being a cooperative patient."

His doctor had told him that surgery would be the next day. So Jim didn't want to offend. He apologized to the nurse, then sank back onto the pillow and tried to relax. Instead he waited and worried, and his stomach churned. A blood transfusion was begun. He watched it drip, drip through the tubing and worried. The next morning his wife was not allowed to see him but everyone else seemed to drop in to do something or promise something. But no one had time to listen to him and he felt more lonely than ever.

Following surgery, Jim completely caved in—he cried and complained constantly. His wife and doctor couldn't understand what had happened.

From the minute Jim entered the hospital, he lost control of his life—he was put in the position of being a child and was told what to do and when to do it. Jim's capacity to reason and his right to dignity were disregarded by almost everyone. When he lashed out at the technician, he stopped being a "good" patient and was punished by the staff. They emotionally abandoned him at the very time when understanding and support were most needed.

Unfortunately, Jim's story is not an unusual one.

Occasionally a hospital patient will try to regain control with some surprising results. One newly admitted patient, for example, was forgotten when the breakfast and lunch trays were passed out. He reminded the nurses that he hadn't received a tray and eventually they brought him one. But when his dinner tray also didn't arrive with the others, the man was so provoked that he put on his clothes and left the hospital. After arriving at a nearby diner, he called the nurses on the floor and told them where he was. "I'll be back after I finish eating." You can bet that the patient got his tray promptly after this incident.

THE FOOD—
LESS THAN NUTRITIOUS

Jokes about hospital food have been standard material for many stand-up comedians and script writers on situation comedies. It's easy to see why—the jokes never grow old.

In pediatric wards across the country, impressionable children receive snacks of canned soda, sweetened and flavored gelatin, and Popsicles. All are loaded with sugar, all are empty calories. Adults in the same hospital are served main dishes made from powdered mixes and frozen meats. These are accompanied by white bread, over-cooked vegetables, canned fruits, and rich desserts. At a time when nourishing meals are most important, sick patients often do not get them.

Here are some familiar examples of how hospitals fail to meet the nutritional needs of their clients:

- Twenty-two-year-old John Myers is recovering from a severe case of pneumonia that has left him weak and anemic. The regular hospital diet does not accommodate his body's increased need for protein and calories. Creamed chicken on toast (where's the chicken?) and paper-thin roast beef are typical entrées.

- Forty-year-old Irene Hammond is recuperating from knee surgery in the local hospital. Accustomed to a diet that includes fresh fruits, vegetables, and whole-grain breads, she has been made constipated by the combination of bland hospital food and lack of exercise. Instead of treating the problem with a high-fiber diet, the physician prescribes pills and bulk laxatives.

- When Joe Merrick was receiving intravenous antibiotic therapy, his gastrointestinal tract was in a turmoil. So why was he served enchiladas with a liberal sprinkling of hot chili powder?

The truth is that the nutritional needs of patients are not clearly understood by hospital personnel, and in the hospital setting, concern for these needs is very low priority.

Additionally, there is often no clear assignment of responsibility. Is the nurse, doctor, or dietician responsible for meeting the patient's nutritional needs? Often, unless a physician orders it, a patient is not apt to have a dietary history taken, and nutritional counseling is not usually provided. There is also a general failure to observe and record the patient's oral food intake, to record height and weight, and to provide vitamin and mineral supplements when necessary.

Numerous studies document the poor nutritional status of many hospitalized patients. Those suffering from alcoholism, eating disorders (obesity, anorexia, or bulimia), anemia, diabetes, food allergies, diarrhea, and other debilitating diseases are particularly vulnerable to malnutrition and would benefit greatly from a customized dietary regime. But regardless of the diagnosis, many patients in the hospital suffer to some degree from inadequate nutrition.

Studies have shown that the levels of certain vitamins and minerals (vitamin C, thiamine, riboflavin, zinc, selenium, and magnesium) fall below the Recommended Dietary Allowances with typical hospital fare. And that's assuming that the patient eats all the food served in a day!

In 1982 the *Alabama Journal of Medical Sciences* suggested that, although malnutrition has often been connected with vitamin deficiency syndromes, these are actually "rare medical curiosities." Protein-calorie malnutrition, on the other hand, is now being recognized in one-fourth to one-half of the medical and surgical patients hospitalized for two weeks or longer.

Whether because of loss of appetite or the effects of disease and/or treatment, many hospitalized patients are malnourished. And patients with protein-calorie malnutrition do not tolerate illness well. They tend to experience delayed wound healing and to have a greater susceptibility to infection and other complications.

AND THE NOISE!

"Dr. Knight, report to labor and delivery STAT . . . Dr. Palmer, paging Dr. Palmer . . ."

At 4:30 A.M., the floor waxer whirs around in the corridor . . .

All day and night, metal bangs against metal on the service elevator . . .

Somewhere in the recesses of the hospital, there's a hammer banging or an alarm clanging . . .

These are some common hospital noises which can add to the tension and anxiety that a patient suffers.

Margaret Topf, PhD, an assistant professor at the University of California at Los Angeles School of Nursing, recently studied noise levels in 27 randomly selected two-, three-, and four-patient rooms at a Veterans Administration hospital. Every two seconds for 24 hours, a special device recorded the number of decibels (db), then tallied the average and maximum sound levels.

The sound levels registered at 55, 54, and 53 for double, triple, and quadruple rooms, respectively, with an overall average of 54.17 db. About 50 percent of the time, noise rose above 50 db.

According to standards set by the Environmental Protection Agency, daily noise exposure in a hospital setting should average no more than 45 db.

Hospitals are *not* peaceful places. At the very time when rest is most important it's impossible for patients to attain, and they suffer because of this.

THERE'S NO QUIBBLING ABOUT COST

If you wanted to have your kitchen remodeled, you would call in a builder for an estimate. But if you went to the hospital to get your upset stomach fixed, not only would you have no idea what the costs would be, but no one would even consult you about these costs. When you think about it, that's a ridiculous way to enter any business arrangement (regardless of whether the government, medical insurance, or you pay the bill). Furthermore, most people don't think in terms of "getting their money's worth" when they're in the hospital. Medicare (using our tax dollars) is willing to pay $3 for a 40¢ razor. Your physician may order $500 worth of tests when $50 worth would give him the same answers.

Health care costs in this country, hovering around 10 percent of the gross national product, have soared out of control. Hospitals account for two-thirds of these costs. According to the American Hospital Association, the average cost for one day in a community hospital is now $463.93 per patient. Paradoxically, as costs continue to rise, the quality of care declines.

In addition, when a patient does receive the hospital bill, it's likely to be full of mistakes. Equifax Services, Inc., of Atlanta, Georgia, which audits hospital bills for major health insurance companies, conducted a survey for 1984. It found that 97 percent of audited hospital bills contained errors.

The firm examined almost 13,000 bills from all 50 states and the District of Columbia and Puerto Rico. These bills averaged $37,834. After they were studied and resubmitted, each was reduced by an average of $1,374.

In this study most billing mistakes were attributed to human error. Laboratory tests and x-rays might have been ordered then canceled, but the charge slip had already been submitted. Data entry errors accounted for other errors. By pressing the wrong key, a $40 charge could have entered the computer as a $400 charge. In the pharmacy department, frequently more medication was ordered than was used.

Some errors in billing can be amusing. One young couple from New York was wading through the hospital bill after their daughter's birth and found an unusual entry. They had been charged for a circumcision!

In a society that prides itself on comparison shopping and customer satisfaction, hospitals just don't measure up to what our expectations should be. Compare, for example, a trip to a luxury resort with a trip to the hometown hospital. By calling my travel agent, I find that a night in one of the swankiest hotel rooms in Las Vegas would run $60 to $100 and a dinner and show would run $32 to

$36. With $463.93 in my pocket (the average cost for one day in a community hospital), I could also enjoy breakfast in bed and a three-course luncheon and still have plenty of money left over to do some shopping or work the slot machines.

Personally, I would prefer the Las Vegas trip, where my world is not limited to the four walls of a dreary hospital room; where I can choose my own roommate; where I can have all the visitors I want and at the time I want them; and where I can dress in something more becoming and distinctive than a skimpy Johnny shirt. To be perfectly honest, I think I'd get a better return for my money if I went to Las Vegas than to my local hospital—I might come back healthier, too.

Chapter 2

WHAT SENDS PEOPLE TO THE HOSPITAL

Many cases can be made for staying *out* of the hospital. Yet the fact still remains that people *do* go to the hospital. Each day, each and every one of the nation's hospitals admits and discharges patients. You could say they do a pretty thriving business. After all, it isn't often that you hear about a hospital shutting down because of a lack of clientele.

In the chart on pages 22–23, you'll find a list of the most common conditions that send people to the hospital. You most likely won't be surprised that births, heart disease, and cancer lead the list. In the following pages I'll discuss these reasons why people go to the hospital and—in some cases—maybe why they shouldn't.

THE HAPPY MOMENT OF BIRTH

Twenty-five years ago, when I was a nursing student, pregnant women received a minimum of prenatal instruction. Neither fathers nor other family members were allowed in the labor or delivery rooms. Mothers were frequently "put to sleep" during birth, and hospital stays lasted five to seven days. But a lot has changed over the years.

Obstetrical care is an area where the medical establishment has responded to consumer activism in a big way.

Today fathers can be active participants during the birth process and delivery, and mothers can experience a more natural labor and delivery. The usual hospital stay has been reduced to three days—some mothers and babies can even leave the hospital the same day the baby is born.

In fact, it's not all that uncommon anymore for a soon-to-be mother to avoid the hospital altogether. There's been a steady increase in the use of nurse-midwives in the past 30 years, and home births have been enjoying a resurgence of popularity. Birthing centers are another alternative that provide some of the best features of both hospital and home birth. (The advantages and disadvantages of these alternatives will be discussed in chapter 5.)

With all the advances in care and caring, obstetrics in the United States today sounds very wonderful until one compares U.S. infant mortality with the rates in other countries:

Country	Infant Mortality per 1,000 Live Births
USA	12
West Germany	13
Britain	12
France	10
Japan	7

With all our technology and know-how, why aren't we doing better? If you look at the chart on pages 22–23, you'll notice that the number of "complicated deliveries" taking place in a hospital setting (where most women still choose to have their children) is greater than the number of "normal deliveries." Simply put, when you go to the hospital to have a baby, you're more likely to experience a complicated birth than a normal one. How can this be? Giving birth is, after all, one of the most "normal" human activities around. So what's the problem?

Malpractice suit is frequently the problem, and in many cases caesarean section—the most common remedy for "complications"— is the solution. This major operation has been increasing steadily in

THE HOSPITAL HIT PARADE

According to the most recent statistics from the National Center for Health Statistics of the United States Public Health Service, the diagnostic category and average length of stay for patients discharged from nonfederal short-stay hospitals is as follows:

Diagnostic Category	Rate per 1,000 Population	Average Length of Stay in Days
Females with deliveries	17.1	3.6
Normal deliveries	7.5	2.8
Complicated deliveries	9.6	4.2
Heart disease	15.5	8.6
Acute myocardial infarction (heart attack)	2.9	10.9
Atherosclerotic heart disease	2.0	8.4
Other ischemic disease	4.0	6.9
Cardiac dysrhythmias	2.0	7.4
Congestive heart failure	2.0	9.7
Malignant neoplasms (cancer)	8.9	10.5
Fractures, all sites	4.7	10.2
Cerebrovascular disease (including stroke)	3.7	11.7

the United States over the past two decades. It is now the third most frequently performed surgery in the country, and often its necessity is debatable. Nowadays, if there's any question of infant distress (as determined by the monitoring machines), a physician most likely will opt to perform a section rather than go through with a vaginal delivery because of its possible risks (no matter how small) and the lawsuit that could result. Also, difficult deliveries (like breech presentations), which formerly would have been done vaginally, are now done by caesarean section.

If fear of medical lawsuits is a big reason for the increase in caesarean sections, it must be pointed out that it is mothers, babies, and fathers who suffer the consequences. At the very least, having a caesarean section is a disappointment to parents, and at the worst it can cause any of the complications that go along with major surgery. It also increases the length of hospital stay for mother and baby, and

Pneumonia, all forms	3.6	8.0
Diabetes mellitus	2.9	9.5
Cataract	2.6	2.5
Arthropathies and related disorders	2.5	8.3
Benign neoplasms, carcinoma in situ, and neoplasms of uncertain behavior	2.5	6.3
Noninfectious enteritis and colitis	2.5	5.1
Psychoses	2.5	15.4
All abortions, including ectopic and molar pregnancies	2.1	2.0
Cholelithiasis	2.1	8.7
Inguinal hernia	2.1	4.1
Asthma	2.0	5.5
Intervetebral disc disorder	2.0	8.2
Diseases of the central nervous system	1.9	10.5
Alcohol-dependence syndrome	1.7	11.5
Chronic disease of tonsils and adenoids	1.7	1.8
All conditions	167.0	6.9

costs more. In addition, no one knows what the long-term effects of caesarean sections are on infants.

Avoiding the Unnecessary

If you're expecting a baby and want to do everything you can to prevent an *unnecessary* caesarean section, I would suggest you discuss the issue very thoroughly with your obstetrician or nurse-midwife. What are the doctor's indications for performing a section? What are the nurse-midwife's criteria for calling in an obstetrician? Are you likely to fall into any of these categories? Not every situation is cut and dried. For example, the old rule of "once a section, always a section" no longer holds true. Some women can have a vaginal delivery after having a caesarean section—it all depends on the reason for the original section.

Many indications for a caesarean section arise during the course of labor and cannot be "planned." But a patient can ask the obstetrician what role the parents have in this decision making. Is it a unilateral decision by the obstetrician or are the parents consulted? If early on the doctor pats you on the head and says, "Don't worry your pretty head about that," you may want to consider finding another obstetrician.

HEART DISEASE KEEPS 'EM BUSY

If you eliminate the "natural experience" of giving birth, the heart of hospital business is treatment of heart disease (it is also this nation's number-one killer).

Acute myocardial infarction is a fancy name for a heart attack, and it almost always sends people to the hospital. But should it?

According to one British report, more patients survive heart attacks if they are treated at home than if they are hospitalized. A team of British physicians compared the records of nearly 2,000 men who experienced heart attacks, half of whom were admitted to the hospital coronary care unit (CCU), the other half of whom were treated at home. At the end of a year, the death rates were 20 percent among patients treated at home and 27 percent for those hospitalized.

In this country it's unlikely that a doctor would recommend that anyone with a severe heart attack remain at home. And it seems that Americans have put so much faith in coronary care units that they think it would be unpatriotic to remain at home. The availability of drugs, oxygen, electrocardiograms, x-rays, and other tests in the hospital makes one feel that the system is "on alert" for any difficulties that may arise.

However, it could be that staying in the hospital for several weeks, hooked up to all the monitors and machinery and being cared for by strangers, may be more stressful—and thus damaging to the patient—than staying at home under medical supervision.

Risk of death from a heart attack is highest within one hour of the onset of the event. Thereafter it falls rapidly. One study found the following percentages: 41.3 percent of deaths occurred between days one and three of hospitalization; 40.3 percent between days four and ten; and 12.4 percent after ten days.

These figures were published in 1976 after a group of cardiologists held a workshop on early hospital discharge of patients with uncomplicated heart attacks. One conclusion of the group was that certain patients can be discharged as early as 7 to 9 days after a heart attack—and perhaps sooner. That recommendation came in 1976, and although average hospital stays have been reduced from 21 to 10.9 days, there's still room for improvement. Ask your doctor—after 2 to 5 days in the hospital coronary care unit and a few days on the medical floor, you may be better off going home.

Should You Bypass the Bypass?

Other types of cardiac treatment that require hospitalization, but that are open to debate, are the increased number of cardiac cathetherizations and coronary bypass operations. In recent years the number of these procedures has reached epidemic proportions. The invasive catheterization test (a risky procedure in which dye is inserted into the arteries, enabling doctors to "see" the extent of damage or artery blockage) can sometimes be replaced by other less hazardous tests, and bypass surgery should be undertaken only after a second opinion confirms its necessity. Although many patients claim that bypass relieves chest pain, it reappears in 40 percent of cases, according to cardiologist Richard Ross, MD, dean of the Johns Hopkins University Medical School. Dr. Ross, in testimony before the Senate Human Resources Subcommittee on Health and Scientific Research, stated: "There is no evidence that the operation prevents sudden death or makes patients with coronary artery disease live longer."

Perhaps you should bypass the popular bypass operation. Medication and change in lifestyle may be just as effective in improving blood flow to the heart—and it'll help keep you out of the hospital.

THE BIG "C"

Although cancer is the second leading cause of death in this country, it is the *number-one* feared disease. The survival rates for many cancers have shown steady improvement because of earlier detection and more effective treatment (stomach and uterine cancers are two examples). In spite of this fact, there is still a public fear that cancer is an automatic death sentence.

It is impossible to speak of *a* treatment for cancer, because cancer is not one disease but a group of over 100 different diseases. And of 50 proven anticancer drugs, no one remedy is effective against more than a few forms of cancer. How treatment is carried out is different too. Skin cancer, for example, is frequently treated on an outpatient basis, but other cancers usually require periods of hospitalization interspersed with home care and use of outpatient services. If the cancer is terminal, a hospice program (discussed in chapter 5) is usually a more humane alternative than acute hospital care.

Where is the best place to receive early cancer treatment? This is an instance where a hospital *is* the best place for the patient to be. But it's the *type* of hospital that's the all-important decision. It is my personal belief that if a patient has a choice, he or she is better off in a large cancer treatment center rather than in a local community hospital. That's because in a cancer center, care is given by health personnel who deal with cancer problems on an everyday basis. That's *all* they do and they're good at it. Another fact: there's often a "lag time" before the successful new therapies given in a cancer center are filtered down and accepted by the local hospital and medical community.

New York City's Memorial Sloan-Kettering Cancer Center is one of the best known and most highly regarded centers in the country. But it's not the only one. In my opinion, it makes sense, after the diagnosis of cancer has been made, to have the treatment program initiated at a cancer treatment center. If this is not possible, there are more than 1,000 hospitals across the country that have cancer programs approved by the Commission on Cancer of the American College of Surgeons. Once the treatment protocol has been established, care can be continued by the local primary care physician at the community hospital if it has the needed radiation and other equipment.

There has been no one definitive study proving that five-year survival rates are improved by obtaining treatment in the larger cancer centers. However, Charles Smart, MD, a surgeon from Salt Lake City, reported significant variations in outcome of cancer care by geographic location. Dr. Smart observed that 468,288 cancer patients treated in cancer programs approved by the American College of Surgeons showed substantial differences in the 15 large geographical areas that were studied. These results showed, for example, that survival for cervical cancer differed by as much as 28 percent. For other cancers (such as Hodgkin's disease, acute leukemia, and melanoma) the differences in rates were 20 percent or more.

Whether the variations in outcome were related to variations in patterns of care is a question that has not been fully answered. One fact is certain: with most cancers, the sooner the diagnosis is made and treatment is begun, the higher the survival rate.

MENDING BROKEN BONES

Remember when you were a kid and you broke your arm, leg, or collarbone (pick one) because you were horsing around with the other kids? Remember what your mother said? It probably went something like this, "If you'd listen to me like you're supposed to, this would never have happened!"

Fractures can happen at any age, and at any age they *can* be avoided, simply by following such sensible safety rules as watching preschoolers more closely, keeping young children out of competitive contact sports until their bodies are in proper condition, buckling up car safety belts, staying off of motorcycles, and avoiding other obviously dangerous situations like riding a skateboard or sky-diving. For the elderly—prone to fractures due to brittle bones—better lighting, hand rails in bathrooms, and the removal of scatter rugs and unnecessary clutter all are useful in preventing dangerous falls.

We aren't always sensible, so we break bones—and wind up in the hospital getting them mended. (After all, after heart disease and cancer, broken bones are the cause of most hospitalizations.)

The usual procedure for a broken bone is to go to the doctor's office or the hospital emergency room, where an x-ray will be taken and the bone will be set.

Hospitalization is seldom necessary unless you have a broken bone that requires an operation, a compound fracture (a bone protruding through the skin) or a fractured skull. Hospitalization is also recommended for those with serious medical problems or those who are very old. In other cases of broken bones, convalescence can take place at home. So don't let a physician persuade you to be admitted simply for *his* convenience.

IT USED TO BE CALLED APOPLEXY

It's estimated that over 500,000 people in the United States have strokes each year. Like a heart attack, it almost always sends them to the hospital.

Because stroke primarily affects the elderly, placement in nursing homes used to be the only choice for most survivors. Yet, in many cases, stroke rehabilitation is a better and more cost-effective alternative to permanent nursing-home care. To many stroke patients it can mean a return to community life and former lifestyle. While at least half of those who survive strokes could benefit from a rehabilitation program, only a small percentage are currently receiving adequate rehabilitative treatment. This is a shame, because in the past two decades tremendous strides have been made in the area of stroke rehabilitation, and the outlook for improving the stroke patient's quality of life is much improved.

Once the diagnosis of a stroke has been made and medical treatment has begun, rehabilitation is the most important concern. In the first 72 hours after a stroke (even the very day of the stroke), physical therapy can begin with proper positioning in bed and range-of-motion exercises. These exercises can be either active (those that the patient does himself) or passive (those that the nurse or therapist helps the patient do), depending on the patient's condition. During these early hours of care, a psychologist or social worker can begin counseling the patient and family. And the dietician can plan the appropriate diet, considering the patient's disability (can the stroke victim swallow?) and medical needs. The speech therapist may make an initial assessment, then make recommendations to staff members and begin family education.

All this work by rehabilitation team members is in addition to the medical care prescribed by the physician in charge and carried out by the nursing staff.

From the third to seventh day after a stroke, when the patient's condition is stabilized, the physical therapist will continue developing a program of exercise and retraining. The rehabilitation nurse will attend to the patient's immediate physical needs but will also, like other team members, be looking to the patient's future in hopes of providing as full a recovery as possible.

Toward the end of the first week following a stroke, the occupational and recreational therapists will begin their assessments and recommendations. The occupational therapist may make a home visit to help the patient and family make necessary household adjustments to assure the patient's safety and independence. The social worker will be looking to the future too. Will rehabilitation training continue on an inpatient or outpatient basis? If home care is desired, will a referral be made to a home health care agency? Will homemaker services or Meals on Wheels be necessary? Could the patient benefit by joining a stroke club or using a day care center?

This is the type of care a stroke patient *should* be getting. If it's not the case, you should find out why or, if it's possible, go to another hospital.

Of course, every stroke patient's rehabilitation program will be different, depending on the patient's age, the severity of the stroke, and other complicating medical problems. Care will also depend on the community facilities that are available and on the support and resources of the family.

A rehabilitation program, which uses the expertise of many disciplines, will provide the very best care for the stroke patient. For those who have a choice, a rehabilitation center is a better alternative than a general hospital, where rehabilitation is not as comprehensive and the chance for full recovery is not as promising.

THOSE BIG— AND LITTLE—SURGERIES

According to the most recent statistics from the National Center for Health Statistics of the United States Public Health Service, the most frequently performed operations for both male and female patients of all ages, who were discharged from nonfederal short-stay hospitals, are:

Surgical Category	Rate per 1,000 Population
Procedures to assist delivery	9.6
Diagnostic dilation and curettage of uterus (D&C)	3.4
Caesarean section	2.7
Hysterectomy	2.7
Bilateral destruction or occlusion of fallopian tubes	2.5
Repair of inguinal hernia	2.3
Cataracts	2.1
with insertion of prosthetic lens	1.1

Besides those listed in the "top seven," other frequently performed surgeries are tonsillectomy, circumcision, gallbladder surgery (cholecystectomy), knee surgery (excision of semilunar cartilage of knee), plastic surgery, and biopsy.

All of these surgeries, except for those connected with the birth of a baby, can be considered "elective," or, in other words, surgery that possibly shouldn't be done at all.

Frequently, the reason for performing surgery in the hospital is that the patient would not receive adequate care at home during the first several postoperative days.

The truth is, however, that many of these procedures—if they *are* necessary—can be carried out in a "surgi-center" or an outpatient surgical clinic instead of a hospital. Home health care or housekeeping services can always be provided for the patient if needed during the postoperative days. (You'll learn all about this in chapter 7.) Those surgeries that can be done outside of the hospital (but aren't always) are dilation and curettage (D&C), tubal ligation (bilateral destruction or occlusion of fallopian tubes), cataract surgery (extraction of lens with or without insertion of prosthetic lens), some hernia repairs, tonsillectomy, some biopsies, and most plastic surgery.

Additionally, knee arthroscopy, vasectomy, and abortion can be performed on an outpatient basis where the stay is shorter, cheaper, more personalized, and there's less chance of picking up an infection. (Outpatient choices are explored in chapter 5.)

In fact, many surgeries that could be done only in the hospital a decade ago are routinely done on an outpatient basis today. So, you'd be best advised to question your options before committing yourself to needless days in the hospital for surgery.

THOSE DIAGNOSTIC TESTS

Also from the Public Health Service are these recent statistics on the most frequently performed diagnostic tests in nonfederal short-stay hospitals (see page 31).

If your doctor recommends that you be admitted to the hospital for *any* diagnostic test, take note. The most frequently performed tests (cystoscopy, radioisotope scan, endoscopy of large intenstine, diagnostic ultrasound, and CAT scan) can all be done on an outpatient basis. So even though it's routinely done, there is no reason (barring extenuating circumstances) why you must be admitted to the hospital to have any of these tests.

Procedure Category	*Rate per 1,000 Population*
Cystoscopy—Examination of the bladder, ureter, and kidney with an instrument called a cystoscope.	3.3
Endoscopy of large intestine—Visual examination of the inside of the large intestine using an instrument called an endoscope.	2.6
Radioisotope scan—Visualization of a radioisotope deposit in an organ using a radiation detector.	2.5
Computerized axial tomography (CAT) scan—Combines x-ray equipment with a computer that analyzes the information and visually reconstructs cross sections of the insides of a body.	2.4
Diagnostic ultrasound—The use of ultrasonic imaging techniques to detect tissue density differences within the body and thus detect disease conditions in various organs. Also used in pregnancy to estimate fetal growth and detect abnormalities.	2.2
Endoscopy of small intestine—Visual examination of the inside of the small intestine using an endoscope.	1.7
Arteriography using contrast material—X-ray of the arteries after injection of a radiopaque substance into the blood vessels.	1.6
Angiocardiography using contrast material—X-ray examination of the blood vessels of the chest and the heart chambers after the injection of radiopaque material into the blood vessels.	1.5
Contrast myelogram—X-ray of the spinal canal, made after the injection of a contrast medium into the space that contains cerebrospinal fluid.	1.4

Endoscopy of the small intestine can usually be done on an outpatient basis too.

Three of the listed procedures (arteriogram or angiogram, cardiac catheterization, and myelogram) can be done on a limited (overnight) inpatient basis.

THOSE SERIOUS MEDICAL PROBLEMS

Diseases of the respiratory system (pneumonia, bronchitis, asthma), gastrointestinal disorders (enteritis, colitis, ulcers of the stomach and small intestine), and metabolic problems (such as diabetes) are frequently treated in the hospital, although the necessity for this is not always clear. For example, only if an ulcer is bleeding or perforated or there are other complications is hospitalization necessary. Present treatment for uncomplicated ulcer can be carried out best on an outpatient basis.

If a patient's illness is potentially life-threatening or if there is an additional medical problem that is complicating treatment, then hospitalization is probably a better alternative than being treated at home. But that doesn't mean a patient should be languishing in the hospital once the initial medical problem has been brought under control. Additional diagnostic tests and treatment can frequently be carried out on an outpatient basis. The story of Joe Merrick in chapter 1 is a perfect example of how staying in the hospital too long can cause unnecessary treatment.

So how long is too long? Modern medicine has no cut-and-dried rules on how long it takes to "cure" a certain condition. People cannot be pigeonholed into various categories and told that their pneumonia will be cured in seven days or ten days. However, in the federal government's desperation to reduce expensive hospitalization for Medicare patients, it *has* pigeonholed patients into 467 disease categories and will pay only a certain amount of money for each ailment. This new process is called the DRG (diagnostic-related groups) system and it's sending hospitals into a tailspin as they try to cut costs and provide more efficient care.

Although it's not certain that DRGs will provide the solution for overhospitalization and spiraling costs, there's no doubt that there is a problem.

You would think, for example, that if physicians and hospitals all use the same basic type of treatment for illnesses, there would be a general uniformity as to how medical care is given across the country. Not so.

By examining the following government statistics on discharges and length of stay for patients in nonfederal short-stay hospitals, according to geographic areas, you can see that you have a greater chance of being hospitalized if you live in the South, but you'll stay in the hospital longer if you live in the Northeast.

Geographic Region	Discharges per 1,000 Population	Average Length of Stay in Days
Northeast	32.5	8.3
North Central	46.4	7.3
South	55.1	6.7
West	26.3	6.0

The best defense for avoiding and cutting your hospital stay is becoming an educated health consumer. That's what this book is all about.

Chapter 3

WHEN THE DOCTOR SAYS, "HOSPITAL!"

Just thinking about it may send chills up your spine. The gray-haired physician, poised and confident, speaks as though he were inviting you to a party. "You'll have to be admitted to the hospital. I'll have my nurse make the necessary arrangements."

With the phrase "admitted to the hospital," your legs turn to rubber and your mind goes numb.

Unlike having a family, going on a dream vacation, or possibly hitting the state lottery, going to the hospital is one of life's events we can miss out on altogether and still go to our grave with the satisfaction that we've done it all.

However, there are times in many people's lives when a hospital is the place—the only place—to be. So, even though this book is about *avoiding* hospitals, it only makes sense to review *all* the situations—hopefully few and far between—when hospitalization is recommended. Some are in your best interest; some may not be to your advantage at all.

THOSE EMERGENCY SITUATIONS

An emergency is defined as "a circumstance demanding immediate action." In terms of your health, that action can mean preventing death or disability.

Generally these situations require ambulance service (or the fastest way of getting to the hospital), emergency room care, and admission to a hospital. Below are some of the situations in which you shouldn't balk (if, in fact, you can talk at all!) when someone screams, "You'd better get to the hospital!"

- *Heart attack*—Fifty percent of all deaths from heart attack occur within 2½ hours of the onset of symptoms. If you are a man over 35 or a woman over 50, you should seek medical care for any chest pain that lasts longer than five minutes. In a heart attack the pain is located behind the breastbone, is described as deep and crushing, and may radiate to the back, the jaw, or the left arm. This is often accompanied by nausea and vomiting, sweating, and shortness of breath. In severe episodes the patient may feel apprehensive or have a sense of impending doom.
- *Severe bleeding*—Bleeding can result from serious trauma and may involve major vessels. Bleeding can also be a factor in perforated ulcers, in which case the vomiting produces bright red or "coffee ground" stained material (or there are black, tarry stools). Severe bleeding from the rectum, the vagina, or the urinary tract also deserves emergency care, as does coughing up blood.
- *Internal injuries*—A penetrating wound to the heart or lungs or rupture of internal abdominal organs demands immediate attention.
- *Breathing problems*—Any unexplained or sudden difficulty breathing (this includes severe allergic reactions) requires prompt medical care.
- *Neurological problems*—Loss of feeling or paralysis of one side of the body, inability to walk, difficulty in speaking or understanding, or sudden loss of vision may be caused by a stroke. Severe headache, convulsions, or loss of consciousness are other serious neurological problems that need prompt evaluation.

- *Accidents*—Severe burns or ingestion of a fast-acting poison requires a trip to the hospital. In addition, any gunshot wound or serious knife wound should be treated in the hospital, and certain fractures (suspected back, neck, or skull fracture or fracture of the extremity where the broken bone protrudes through the skin) also require immediate hospital care.
- *Acute psychiatric problems*—A person who has experienced a sudden and complete change in personality needs immediate care.

In *any* emergency situation you and your family have the right to be fully informed. You should be told what your diagnosis is; what test, treatment, or surgery is recommended; and what the alternatives are. If you are experiencing a life-threatening problem, such as those listed, you should be seen immediately on your arrival at the hospital by an emergency room physician.

Be Prepared!

Although you may not be able to prevent the actual occurrence of an emergency problem, you *can* plan ahead with your physician and family so that *everything* isn't left to chance.

For example, do you know right now what steps you would take if an emergency arose? Do you know the emergency number to call? Is it posted near your telephone? Do you know who will respond when that number is called?

If you live in a district that has a paramedic program, you will receive immediate emergency care. Using information received from the paramedic, a certified mobile intensive care nurse (MICN)—located at a base-station hospital—will evaluate your condition and follow a certain protocol in prescribing treatment that the paramedic can administer at the scene and en route to the hospital. The emergency room physician will also be available to give advice by radio transmission. This situation usually brings the fastest and best emergency care to your doorstep. But if you don't live in a paramedic district, a fireman or private ambulance service or even a policeman could respond to your call. However, they may or may not have emergency training, and the response time may be slow.

Regardless of the services your community offers, it's important for every person to be proficient in administering CPR (cardiopulmonary resuscitation) and to have basic first-aid skills. The American Red Cross offers classes in both areas, and the American Heart Association gives a course in CPR.

Next, do you know which hospital emergency room you will go to in case of serious illness or injury? Is there a doctor available 24 hours a day in this hospital or does a doctor need to be called when an emergency arises at night? It's best if there is a doctor present at all times. Are the emergency doctors board certified in such specialities as emergency medicine, family practice, or internal medicine? To some professionals this is an important criterion for judging quality of care. To others, the most important criterion is experience. If you go to a medical center emergency room, are the interns and residents supervised by a physician experienced in emergency medicine? In any hospital, are the emergency room nurses certified in advanced cardiac life support? They should be.

Does the hospital near your home have an intensive care unit or a coronary care unit? If it doesn't, would you have a choice of hospitals to which you could be transferred? What are the reputations of these hospitals?

If it's possible, you should have two people go with you to the emergency room or, if you are being transported by an ambulance, have them meet you there. One would talk with the staff and serve as your spokesperson—the other would stay by your side. Both people should know something of your health history, previous surgeries, and your present medical problem. They should know the name of your private physician and what medications you are taking (bring bottles if not sure of names—especially if drug overdose is a factor in the emergency).

Finally, your family and physician should know your feelings on heroic measures to prolong life and should know if you've made out a living will. A living will is a legal document that specifies the treatment you want or don't want if you become critically ill and have no reasonable expectation of recovery. The hospitalized patient who is comatose, for example, is no longer able to express his or her desires, but could make these wishes known ahead of time by making out a living will. This document might ask that in a hopeless situation no extraordinary measures be taken, such as calling a code (to restore breathing and heartbeat) or keeping a patient on a ventilator or a kidney dialysis machine.

Originally, living wills had no legal power, but in 1976 California passed the first "natural-death act," legally recognizing living wills drafted according to certain requirements. Since then, most states and the District of Columbia have enacted similar legislation.

If you're considering preparing your own living will, it would be best to consult an attorney so that you can find out what the law is in your state, and what must be included in the will to make it valid. In states without natural-death laws, you may use a standardized form or have your attorney design one (you may obtain forms from the Society for the Right to Die, a not-for-profit organization located at 250 West 57th Street, New York, NY 10107. The organization also publishes a book, *Handbook of Living Will Laws, 1981–1984,* available for a fee.)

Once your living will is prepared, give copies to your family and your doctor, and if you're admitted to the hospital, ask that a copy be placed in your medical record.

THOSE SERIOUS MEDICAL PROBLEMS

Doris Smith, 55, has been a diabetic for 15 years. The diagnosis was made when her sixth (and last) baby was born. In spite of her chronic illness, however, Doris lives her life much like anyone else her age. She has no difficulty administering her daily insulin, following her prescribed diet, or testing her urine for sugar. She sees her doctor regularly.

A proud grandmother, Mrs. Smith was baby-sitting for her youngest grandson, Brent, one afternoon and watched the little guy scoot around the living room on all fours. Brent stopped to examine a light cord and put the cord in his mouth. Mrs. Smith jumped up from the couch and ran across the room to rescue Brent. In the process, the grandmother banged her stockinged foot on the coffee table. But it didn't hurt and she was so concerned with her grandson's safety that she didn't even consider her foot until the next day, when she noticed that her big toe had been cut slightly and was black and blue. She washed the foot and applied lanolin. Then she pushed the whole matter to the back of her mind and spent time with her house guests, especially her little guy Brent.

Some days later the foot was painful, cold, and numb. An ulcer was forming. Doris saw her family doctor and he recommended immediate hospitalization. Besides the possibility of gangrene in her foot, Doris's diabetes was out of control. The doctor, whom Doris had known for 20 years, spelled all this out for her. Once she was in the hospital, an endocrinologist was called in, and Mrs. Smith's care was closely monitored by the new specialist.

Few people could quarrel with Doris Smith's need for hospitalization, although at the time of admission her life was in no immediate danger. A stubbed toe doesn't normally send people to the hospital, but because Doris was a diabetic, the injury was complicated by her condition. The careful monitoring that she received in the acute care setting was crucial to her recovery.

The same can be said of patients who suffer from other serious chronic conditions (like emphysema, heart disease, or cancer) when there's a sudden deterioration in that condition. Other serious problems that usually require hospitalization are major surgical operations or major catheterization procedures, such as heart or major blood vessel catherization.

In cases such as these, acute care hospitalization is the best (and sometimes the only) alternative. But here again it helps to have a primary care physician who can make this judgment (taking into account all the variables of your illness, your attitude on hospitalization, and your lifestyle). He should be able to plan events so that you're in and out of the hospital as quickly as possible. In addition, your primary care physician should be able to coordinate the specialists who see you and get action when no one else can. That's because the specialists depend on your primary care physician to refer patients to them.

THOSE
ELECTIVE SURGICAL OPERATIONS

This is the gray area: surgery than can wait a week or more. Sometimes elective surgery is the surgery that should *never* be done.

The story goes something like this:

You're 50 years old, a little overweight maybe, but generally in good health. You go out to dinner one night and overindulge in all sorts of wonderful—but heavy—food. The next day you're suffering—your stomach is queasy and you have gas pains. The incident passes. The next week it's another heavy meal and more troubles. This time the pain seems to be focused on the right side of the abdomen, just below your ribs and it spreads to your chest and back. A well-meaning friend suggests a "gallstone attack" (her sister had trouble for years). Your friend's concern translates into anxiety for you. The pain becomes unbearable.

You see your family physician and he recommends x-ray examination of the gallbladder. Sure enough: gallstones (it's been estimated that 10 percent of American men and 20 percent of American women between the ages of 55 and 60 have gallstones). So now you see the surgeon and he concurs: the gallbladder must go. "You should have the surgery now while you're still young—while you're in good health—while you're not vomiting and dehydrated from a severe attack."

Do you have a choice? You go for it.

Two weeks later you're on the operating table. Your hospital stay is a trial, and the recuperative period at home is long. A year after surgery you still have difficulty digesting fatty foods.

Twenty-five million operations are performed every year in this country—one operation for every ten people. Most can be justified—many cannot. There are certain nonemergency surgeries that may not be necessary, in other words the benefits may not balance out the risks that patients take in having the procedures done. These operations are:

- Gallbladder surgery (cholecystectomy)
- Hysterectomy
- Back surgery (disk surgery)
- Hernia repair
- Hemorrhoid surgery
- Mastectomy
- Tonsillectomy
- Knee joint surgery
- Caesarean section
- D&C (diagnostic dilation and curettage of uterus)
- Coronary bypass surgery
- Sterilization operations (tubal ligation and vasectomy)
- Cataract surgery

This is not a complete list. There's also surgery for ulcers and other gastrointestinal disorders, surgery for stroke patients, arthritics, patients with thyroid and varicose vein problems, and surgery for those who suffer from impotence and obesity. There are all manner of plastic and cosmetic surgeries as well as a number of invasive tests that are almost as hazardous as surgery.

It's not within the scope of this book to delve into all the indications, complications, and alternatives to such procedures. There are, however, some excellent books on the market that do just that. A few are:

Editors of *Prevention* magazine. *The Prevention Guide to Surgery and Its Alternatives.* Emmaus, Pa.: Rodale Press, 1980.

Kra, Siegfried J., and Robert S. Boltax. *Is Surgery Necessary?* New York: Macmillan Publishing Co., 1981.

Schneider, Robert G. *When to Say No to Surgery.* Englewood Cliffs, N.J.: Prentice-Hall, 1982.

BEWARE OF SURGICAL "EPIDEMICS"

Your chances of having certain operations varies statistically according to your age and sex. It also varies according to where you live.

For more than a decade, John Wennberg, MD, professor of epidemiology at Dartmouth Medical School, has been examining the rate of surgery and other forms of medical treatment in 193 small areas in the six New England states. In one city in Maine the rate of hysterectomy was so high that if the rate persisted, 70 percent of the women there would have had the operation by age 75. In a city less than 120 miles away, the rate of hysterectomy was at a level that if it continued, only 25 percent of the women would have had the operation by the time they were 75.

In an area of Vermont the tonsillectomy rate over a four-year stretch was such that if it remained the same, 60 percent of all children would have had their tonsils removed by age 20. In another Vermont area only 8 percent would have had their tonsils removed by age 20. In the area with fewer tonsillectomies, however, the prostatectomy rate was so high that 59 percent of all men would have had their prostate gland removed by age 80. In an area nearby, only 15 percent would have had a prostatectomy by age 80.

Such great differences in the rate of surgery were not observed for a few other common surgical procedures, largely because physicians agree on the need for the operation. But most rates are highly variable. Dr. Wennberg is of the opinion that these "variations occur because there is no consensus about the best procedures." He believes that the "scientific basis of medicine is less well developed than conventional wisdom would have us believe."

So what action does Dr. Wennberg suggest for stabilizing surgical rates? Educating the 500,000 American physicians about the extent of medical variations in their own communities. The profession, he says, should attempt to change these variations through the education and cooperation of physicians. Dr. Wennberg's plan also calls for broad-based support from patients, community leaders, business and labor groups, and government.

Other studies also have confirmed the fact that surgical rates vary from area to area. But is the variation really due to lack of education and consensus by different physicians? Of equal importance, in the view of many, is the supply of specialists in the area. Specialists—like any other business people—will create a market for their services. If there are more cardiovascular surgeons, more coronary bypass surgery will be done. If there are more gynecologists, more hysterectomies will be done, and so on.

And then there's the issue of patient demand. Some patients insist on the quick surgical "cure" rather than accept a long-term medical regime that may require some inconvenience or even a change in lifestyle. Also, some patients have a low tolerance for pain and some, quite frankly, enjoy the whole business of surgery and hospitalization and will jump at the chance to get attention this way (particularly if someone else is paying for it).

GET THE FACTS STRAIGHT

Let's get back to the individual patient who has just been told, for example, that she "needs" a hysterectomy. She is not thrilled at the news. She is not interested in going to the hospital, having the surgery, and suffering through all the postsurgical problems if the operation is not even necessary. She may know that a hysterectomy is one of those surgeries that has a high variation rate, so she is justifiably skeptical. It would help if she knew whether the surgeon who recommended the surgery has a high rate of hysterectomies (compared with other gynecologists) and if the community in which she lives has a high or low rate compared with other communities of equal size, socioeconomic level, and so on.

It would be nice if such information were readily available to patients in every community across the country. Unfortunately, this is not yet the case (although with the rise of consumer activism, it's only a matter of time before this information will be available).

In the meantime, what's a prospective surgical patient to do? Some suggestions:

1. *Change* your *attitude*—The media blasts out the DANGER SIGNS and you're urged to see your physician IMMEDIATE-LY. So you rush to the doctor at the first twinge, ache, or pain. In your anxiety you may exaggerate things a tad and so the doctor orders the x-ray, writes the prescription, or makes the referral. Maybe your physician is thinking lawsuit, maybe he just wants you to be satisfied. But for whatever reason, your concern and anxiety translate into action that may not be necessary and may even be dangerous.

If you see even a little of yourself here, try to have more faith in your body's ability to right itself rather than modern medicine's ability to perform miracles. Also, be informed as to what is and is not a serious symptom or situation.

2. *Realistic versus unrealistic expectations*—On TV you're assured of "overnight relief," "100 percent guarantees," and "immediate satisfaction." In real life, however, there are few magic potions. And as a person gets older, there are fewer "cures"—it's maintenance. So the problems that are easily fixed at age 20 may have to be accepted at age 70. That's a fact of life.

3. *Ask lots of questions*—If surgery is recommended for you, you should ask the following questions (and receive answers that satisfy you).

What is my problem?

What caused it?

What is the expected outcome of the proposed surgery?

What are the risks involved? How likely are they to occur?

Are there alternatives to surgery? What are they?

What is the approximate length of the hospital stay?

Can the surgeon "walk through" the procedure with me so I know what tests and treatments will be done prior to surgery and what will happen in surgery?

What condition will I be in following the operation?

How long will the post-hospital recuperative period be?

What changes in lifestyle will be necessary during this period?

When can normal activities be resumed?

What are the costs of the operation?

Will my insurance cover all the costs?

It's surprising how many people will leave the surgeon's office knowing that an operation is necessary but not knowing what's wrong with them or any of the other facts that concern *their body*. How can this happen?

To begin with, once the specialist says, "I recommend surgery," many patients go deaf and dumb. All those things they "should have said" are totally forgotten. Fear, shock, anger—these are some of the feelings that block logical thinking.

In addition, the body language of many specialists says, "Hurry, hurry, hurry." The surgeon may glance at his watch, tap his fingers, or dash off a few notes and close your chart. As the doctor walks out the door, he may glance over his shoulder and ask, "Any questions?" There's hardly time to say good-by before he's down the hall seeing the next patient.

So, under these circumstances, how can a patient get the facts?

Go to the doctor's office prepared. If it will help, copy the above list of questions (and add your own). If surgery is recommended, pull out your questions and, if necessary, write down the answers. If the doctor is too busy to answer your questions, tell him you can call him later. If he says not to worry about the details of your surgery, then find another doctor who *will* answer your questions.

If you're too upset at the time of the visit to ask questions, ask the surgeon or nurse if you can call at a time that is convenient for him. If you're afraid to ask a "dumb" question, ask the nurse. Nurses are always asked "dumb" questions (except there's no such thing as a "dumb" question).

4. *See your family doctor first*—Having a regular primary care physician will go a long way in eliminating even the question of surgery. Your primary care physician, if he's acting in *your* interest (and he should be) may wait and see or try an alternative medical approach before referring you to a surgeon. Always remember that surgeons *like* to operate much as truck drivers like to drive and painters like to paint. Once you walk into the surgeon's office, you've already made a significant step on the way to the operating room. So it's best to have a primary care physician who'll keep you healthy and try other nonsurgical approaches first.

Second, if your primary care physician refers you to a surgeon and the recommendation is to operate, then you can go back—comfortably—to your primary care physician and discuss the whole issue with him. Can he give you the hard facts on risks and alternative treatments (that you may have forgotten to ask the surgeon about)? Can he refer you to another surgeon?

5. *Get a second opinion*—Because there are differences of opinion among doctors as to whether nonemergency surgery should be done, it makes sense to get more than one opinion. It not only makes sense—it's crucial.

Many insurance companies now offer the option of getting another opinion. In Minnesota, employees of the state and the state university who subscribe to Blue Cross and Blue Shield *must* obtain a second opinion before elective surgery or the insurer won't pay. In addition, the second opinion must come from a physician approved by the insurer who pays for it. If the second physician disagrees with the first, Blue Cross and Blue Shield will pay for a third opinion, including any tests ordered by the physician.

Since April 1, 1983, the New York State Health Insurance Program has required that all active enrollees (and retired enrollees residing in New York State) *must* arrange a second opinion through the State Surgical Consultation Program for the following elective procedures, in order to receive normal plan benefits in excess of the annual deductible:

Bunionectomy	Hysterectomy
Cataract removal	Knee surgery
Deviated septum repair	Prostatectomy

In cases where such elective surgery is performed without a second opinion through the state's second surgical consultation program, benefits will be paid to 50 percent of covered hospital expenses and 50 percent of covered medical/surgical expenses in excess of the annual deductible.

Other insurance plans are also getting on the second-opinion bandwagon. But to many patients, seeking another opinion is an inconvenience that they have neither the time nor interest to pursue. But according to Herbert Denenberg, consumer watchdog and former Pennsylvania insurance commissioner, studies indicate that second opinions reduce the number of operations performed by as much as 20 to 60 percent.

Getting a second opinion is now standard medical practice. For one patient the process went like this:

Five-year-old Johnny is seen by his pediatrician, who recommends that Johnny's mother take the boy to an ear, nose, and throat specialist. The pediatrician has been treating Johnny for repeated tonsillitis, and in his judgment it's time for the tonsils to be surgically removed. One week later, Johnny is seen by the specialist that his pediatrician recommended. In the opinion of the ear, nose, and throat doctor, a tonsillectomy should be done. But Johnny's mother is not sure, so she contacts her health insurer and gets the name of another specialist. She fills out a form and this is sent to the first specialist, who sends Johnny's history and lab test results to the new specialist who will furnish the second opinion. The second specialist knows he will not be performing the surgery but examines Johnny and recommends that surgery be delayed. At this point Johnny's mother could seek still another opinion, go back to Johnny's pediatrician and discuss the whole matter again, have the surgery done out of pocket (if the insurance company won't pay), or wait and see. But the final decision for surgery definitely rests squarely on the shoulders of Johnny's parents. That's because a tonsillectomy is an elective, controversial surgery that has its promoters and detractors.

In Johnny's situation the insurance carrier provided Johnny's mother with a list of specialists who render second opinions. If you don't have this option, you may obtain a second opinion in a number of other ways:

- Ask the first specialist if he could give you the name of another doctor who treats patients with your problem. On the surface, this may seem to be the easiest approach, but it's not necessarily the best one. If the specialists are friends, you may get a less than objective second opinion.
- Contact the local medical society or medical schools in your community for the names of doctors who specialize in the field in which your illness falls. You can then "check out" the prospective specialist in the *Directory of Medical Specialists* (available in most large libraries) to be sure the doctor is board certified.
- Call the HEW toll-free number, 1-800-638-6833 (in Maryland, call 1-800-492-6603) to locate a specialist in your community.
- If you are covered by Medicare, call your local Social Security

office (listed in the telephone directory under U.S. Government, Department of Health, Education, and Welfare).
- If you are eligible for Medicaid, call your local welfare office.

Occasionally, a patient finds that a specialist is less than excited to give an opinion on a case for which he will have no further responsibility. The office secretary may say that the surgeon never questions a colleague's diagnosis and will not render a second opinion. Or the secretary may say that a patient must be referred by another doctor (rather than the patient calling directly) in order to get another opinion. Certainly it's the privilege of any doctor to refuse to see a patient. It's also best for a patient to be candid about the reason he or she is seeing the specialist, saying something like, "I'd like to be examined by Dr. X and see what he finds. If it's necessary to have surgery, Dr. Y will be doing it." Since the physician is being paid for his expert opinion, there is no reason why *you* should feel intimidated by any doctor.

Getting a second opinion is a right that you have as a patient. It can help you make a better, more informed decision about surgery. It can reassure you that surgery is necessary or, if it's not necessary, it can save you time, money, pain, and inconvenience. It can also save your life.

OH, MY ACHING BACK!

If you're still not convinced that seeking a second opinion is worth the time and trouble, I offer the following story.

In 1963, while working as a public health nurse in upstate New York, I was in an automobile accident and injured my back. Another nurse from the health department took me to the local hospital. After the emergency room physician diagnosed the problem as a slipped disk, my co-worker said sympathetically, "I hope you won't need surgery, but usually that's what happens. These things just don't get better without it."

Surgery? No way!

In a flash I remembered my movie idol of the 1950s—Jeff Chandler. I remembered his "he-man" appeal and his cool strength as Cochise in *Broken Arrow*. I also remembered reading the *New*

York Times account of his death (June 18, 1961):

"Jeff Chandler, the movie actor, died of blood poisoning following spinal surgery. He was 42 years old."

"Mr. Chandler, who underwent three operations, was hospitalized May 13 for correction of a slipped spinal disk. Five days later, he experienced severe abdominal bleeding."

I was a third-year nursing student at the time of Chandler's death. Although I never found out the whole story of the actor's demise, I was able to piece together a few more facts by reading other newspaper accounts.

Chandler entered Culver City Hospital (near Los Angeles) on May 13 and surgery was performed for a slipped disk. Five days later he experienced severe abdominal bleeding and was rushed to the operating room. Surgeons kept him alive in a 7½-hour operation during which they administered 55 pints of blood. On May 27 new bleeding broke out and doctors operated again. His condition became weaker after a disheartening series of relapses, including an infection.

"He seemed to be rallying," a spokesman reported, "but his condition became worse Friday."

On Saturday, June 18, his former wife, two children, and his parents were summoned to the hospital. He died that day.

And so here I was, two years later, vowing to myself that I would never have surgery for *my* back problem. And I didn't. The ER physician referred me to a conservative orthopedist who recommended neither hospitalization nor surgery. Instead, he prescribed bed rest, aspirin, crutches, a back brace, and several months of physical therapy before considering a more extreme approach. Convalescence was not easy but the back problem did resolve itself and, more important, I learned many techniques from the physical therapist that have helped to prevent additional back problems (among them were abdominal muscle-strengthening exercises).

I was lucky. I know that a slipped disk can't kill you, but the surgery for it can. And yet every year 250,000 people in this country undergo surgery for a slipped disk. In spite of the fact that surgeons will tell their patients that this operation carries a very low risk, that's small comfort if you or a family member succumb. And don't assume that you will necessarily feel better following this type of surgery. Quite the contrary, you may very well feel worse.

Since a slipped disk presses against nerves that serve the back and legs, serious neurological problems *may* result that necessitate surgery. However, surgery is said to be justified as a treatment for only 1 percent of all who suffer low-back pain. So permanent neurological damage is not the usual reason for doing the $10,000 disk operation. The usual reason is the pain and inconvenience that disk problems cause. But is this reason enough? I'm not sure. In the "old days," when patients suffered from a slipped disk, the prescription was bed rest and supportive treatment. Maybe it's time to return to such simple, less invasive measures.

Certainly it's appropriate to get a second opinion when the question of surgery arises. If Jeff Chandler were alive today, I'm sure he would agree.

Chapter 4

WHAT YOUR DOCTOR CAN DO FOR YOU

Norman Cousins, author of *Anatomy of an Illness* and senior lecturer at the University of California at Los Angeles Medical School, treated his spinal arthritis by using a number of unorthodox methods. Cousins gives primary credit for the successful treatment to his physician. Writing in *Time* magazine (Letters to the Editor, July 15, 1985), Cousins said, "My doctor encouraged me to believe I was a respected partner in the program of recovery, and he recognized the importance of the patient's own psychological resources. Nothing was done that did not have his full support. I agree that attitudes are no substitute for competent medical attention, but confidence in oneself and in the doctor can help create an environment in which medical science can do its best."

More and more, patients are realizing the importance of having a satisfactory relationship with that trusted servant you familiarly call your family doctor.

Your family doctor can be perceived as the general who keeps the troops in line or the traffic controller who keeps all systems running smoothly. He or she can also be your ally in keeping you out of the hospital.

What exactly can your doctor do for you? He can, on a regular basis, oversee your usual health needs and stay attuned to your particular family situation and your lifestyle. Unlike some over-trained specialists, your family doctor can look for the usual rather than the bizarre diagnosis. If a specialist is needed, he can recommend and refer. In a time of emergency, your doctor can be the familiar face that gets the system moving.

When my parents were growing up, the general practitioner (as they were then called) was the person to whom you brought all your medical problems. He was a jack-of-all-trades—treating medical problems, delivering babies, setting bones, and performing surgery. He was a family caretaker in every sense of the word. However, as medical care became more complex and hospitals put restrictions on what doctors could do, the concept of a general practitioner seemed as outdated as the horse and buggy that he drove. The age of specialization had arrived.

Now another trend has emerged—the popularity of the "primary care physician." Other titles for this health worker are general internist, primary care internist, family practitioner, or family physician. For children and young adults, it might be a pediatrician or a specialist in adolescent medicine.

As much as these are deemed "specialties" (in 1970 the American Board of Family Practice offered its first certifying examinations), the role of a primary care physician is that of a generalist. This is the doctor you see for common medical problems and he is your guide to other medical care. He is your protector against unnecessary procedures and your adviser on how you can have a healthy lifestyle.

GETTING TO KNOW YOU

You're indeed fortunate if you can establish a long-term relationship with a competent primary care physician. It can be cheaper for you, and you'll be less likely to have unnecessary surgery or treatments.

However, there are some problems. Not enough physicians are going into this specialty because it does not have the status or draw the salary that other specialties do. According to the American Medical Association, the number of specialists in family practice, pediatrics, and general practice rank third, fourth, and seventh, respectively, in this country. The two specialties with the most practicing physicians are within the broad field of internal medicine (such as endocrinology or cardiology) and general surgery.

In addition, there may not be much excitement in treating a common cold or sprained ankle when a physician has struggled through four years of college, four years of medical school, and additional years of training in a specialty. Many physicians feel that they are overtrained for these routine medical problems. And so other personnel are "filling the gaps" in providing primary health care.

These others are mainly nurse practitioners and physician assistants. (Although these workers provide only the routine and less critical care and work under the supervision of a physician, there is some reluctance on the part of the medical establishment to accept their role. It would seem that some family practitioners don't want to care for minor medical problems—especially in certain segments of the population—but they don't want anyone else to do it either.)

A physician assistant or nurse practitioner can function adequately for most routine problems and will probably spend more time listening and offering health advice than a physician would. But when your medical problems get complicated or you need the extra clout that is necessary in the hospital setting, a primary care physician is your best bet.

Another health worker who often functions as a primary care provider for women is the obstetrician-gynecologist. Because many women understand the importance of regular breast exams and Pap tests, the ob-gyn is the one they visit regularly for health care. For general medical problems, however, the ob-gyn's care is not up to par with that of the primary care physician. And calling in an ob-gyn to coordinate your care when you arrive in the emergency room might raise a few eyebrows among the staff.

But obstetrician-gynecologists are not the only specialists who frequently take on the job of primary care physician. A recent article in the *Journal of the American Medical Association (JAMA)* pointed out that because of an oversupply of neurologists in this country, "their role has changed from that of a consultant for the more difficult problems encountered in practice to that of a physician whose scope of professional activity expands to include the common, self-limited neurological disorders." Specifically, it seems that neurologists are spending half their time treating cases of migraine, severe headaches, and backaches—common conditions that might better be left to the primary care physician. As a result of this trend, many neurologists are in a competitive rather than a consultative relationship with the family doctor.

Furthermore, according to the *JAMA* article, "the cost of the primary care provided by specialists is greater than that provided by primary care physicians, without evidence of improvement in the quality of physician performance."

So having a competent primary care physician who treats most of your medical problems is more efficient, less confusing, less expensive, and in most cases, as "safe" as seeing a different specialist at every turn.

SELECTING A PRIMARY CARE PHYSICIAN

How do you choose a primary care physician? Carefully. Shop around for your doctor as you would any other consumer service, using the following criteria:

Search for Competence

You can find out about a physician's training and expertise by several methods. You can call the physician's office, the hospital, or the county or state medical society to find out where your potential doctor earned his medical degree. You can also go to the library and look up your doctor in the American Medical Association's *Directory of Physicians* or the *Directory of Medical Specialists*. You can find such information as when your doctor was born, when and where he attended medical school and when be became licensed in the state, and whether he's certified in a particular specialty.

Another measure of a doctor's competence is his affiliation with a reputable hospital. In good hospitals there are certain controls placed on physicians by their peers. Although the system is not perfect, association with a top-notch hospital is a good recommendation.

Finally, you can ask around in the medical community about the reputation of the physician you're considering. Other doctors, nurses, or pharmacists are possibilities. Or you can contact your county medical society. Reputation among patients, however, may not be a good gauge of quality because each person's taste and criteria are so different.

The "Right" Chemistry

Do you prefer a doctor who is technically "top notch"—the best in the field—who is also the silent authority figure? Or do you like the "people person" who will be warm and caring, who will listen to your troubles and be a good interpreter of medical jargon?

When you first meet, does the doctor's style and manner meet your expectations and do you trust him?

Is it important to you to have a doctor of your same sex, or one who shares a similar ethnic, racial, or religious background? A doctor with a similar background could possibly understand your feelings and family situation better.

And then there's the matter of age. If you are young and looking for a long-term relationship with a doctor, it might make sense to select a young person. A young doctor, fresh out of school and residency, will probably be up on all the latest techniques. But although the young doctor may be *smart,* he may not be *wise.* Experience is a wonderful teacher, and much is gained after years of handling many different situations.

But then again, an older doctor may have such a busy practice that he would not always be available when needed.

Young versus old: It's not an open-and-shut case. Selecting your doctor is a personal matter that requires considerable thought and investigation. Don't shortchange yourself by accepting a situation that will cause you frustration and anger.

Establishing Rapport

Webster's Dictionary describes rapport as, "a close or sympathetic relationship; agreement; harmony."

A person can usually tell pretty quickly if a doctor is going to be one with whom he or she could establish rapport. In such a personal decision, of course, certain qualities may be more important to one person than to another. However, there are a few guidelines that may help in determining if a certain doctor would be a good "fit" for you.

Because physicians make diagnoses and because history taking is crucial to making those diagnoses, it is imperative that your doctor be able to ask you pertinent questions and that he be able to understand your answers. But if a doctor doesn't speak the same language as you do (and there are many foreign-born physicians in this country), or the doctor mumbles, or is hard of hearing, or is so shy that communication is difficult, you could have problems in establishing rapport.

Beyond the spoken word, does the physician's body language say that he cares about you as a person, or that he sees you as just another "case"? For example, does the physician look you in the eye when talking with you and, when in the office, does he give you his undivided attention or does he take phone calls or diddle with things on his desk? Does the doctor take your problems seriously or does he always make you feel like your illness is not significant or not worthy of his time? Can you ask questions of the doctor? Does he answer those questions fully or does he offer a patronizing, "You don't need to know that" or "It's too complicated—you wouldn't understand." Does the doctor encourage you to write down questions at home (as they occur to you) and bring them to the office with you? If he really cares about you, he should.

Finally, do you think that the physician in question can keep a confidence, or do you feel that telling your troubles to him or to his nurse would be like telling a gossip columnist? Does the physician you're considering espouse positive health practices even though he's overweight or smokes or has poor personal hygiene?

Paul Sanazaro, MD, professor of medicine at the University of California at San Francisco, conducted a telephone survey of 200 patients who were receiving continuing medical care for common chronic conditions.

Almost 90 percent of those surveyed said they were satisfied with their physicians' explanations, but only 58 percent actually had a good understanding of their condition. And 31 percent stated they did not expect their doctor "to treat them as a person." It seems that many physicians have a ways to go.

A Matter of Convenience

Is the doctor's office located near your home and are office hours convenient? Can you get an appointment fairly quickly and are you seen within a reasonable time? When you call the doctor with a significant question, do you receive a prompt answer?

A physician who continually puts his time and convenience before yours is not worth the aggravation. Find someone else who will respect your rights.

The Personal Touch

A doctor's office should appear clean and well equipped, and the office personnel should be pleasant and helpful.

When you make an office visit, the competent physician should listen to your complaints and should perform a careful physical examination. You should be skeptical if a physician recommends a costly treatment for a problem that you're not aware of.

You should be wary if the doctor *constantly* puts an emphasis on the newest drugs or the newest treatments. These may not have stood the test of time.

The Question of Cost

The doctor should be willing to discuss fees and should accept your financial situation and method of payment.

You should be concerned if a doctor continually refers you to other specialists (especially if the problems are of a minor nature), as this will run up your bills.

Your doctor should prescribe generic drugs whenever possible, since this will save you money.

Just a few years back, it would have seemed unreasonable that a patient could "hire and fire" a doctor. Patients often felt fortunate just to get an appointment with someone who carried the intimidating MD initials after his name. Patients frequently put physicians in godlike positions and talked of not wanting to "waste the doctor's valuable time."

Nowadays, some folks condemn the medical profession at every turn and are glad for the bad press and lawsuits that occur.

Actually, neither approach is very healthy. The best relationship between doctor and patient should lie somewhere between trust and skepticism. Medical services are consumer services, and patients should be satisfied with their doctor's performance or find another doctor.

It is being predicted that there will be an oversupply of all physicians in the next decade. What this may mean is that doctors will have to answer patients' needs or they will not be able to make a living. Doctors will have to do things they haven't done in a long time, like listening to their patients, spending time with them, and even making house calls.

Chapter 5

QUALITY & CARE— THE NONHOSPITAL SETTING

- The carpenter's hand slips as he saws a board and the jagged-edged tool puts a nasty gash in his left thumb. As painful as the cut is, even more bothersome is the thought that one of his co-workers will have to drive him across town to a hospital emergency room. The waiting and the hassle will take hours, and with production already behind schedule, the boss will not be happy to lose two workers for that period of time. It's a dilemma that's all too common.
- Two-year-old Jody wakes from her nap with a fever and complains of an earache. At 4 P.M., being "fitted in" at the pediatrician's office is out of the question. Being seen at the emergency room in less than two hours and for less than $100 is also out of the question. So what's a mother to do?
- It's Saturday afternoon and 17-year-old Randy has twisted his ankle in a league softball game. The coach wants to take him to the emergency room to "check it out." But just the thought of wasting the rest of his Saturday at the local hospital is more than Randy can bear.

If these patients lived in Escondido, California, just north of San Diego (or in many other places across the country), they could go to the Emergency Medical Doctors Center located in a downtown shopping center. The facility is open from 8 A.M. to 8 P.M. seven days a week. Without an appointment the carpenter could have his cut cleaned and closed with stitches, get a tetanus booster, and be back on the job in an hour's time. The two-year-old and her mother could walk into the center, be seen by a doctor, and leave—with a prescription for an antibiotic in hand—in less than a half-hour. The young athlete could also receive traditional care in a reasonable period of time at a cost comparable to a doctor's office visit but at less than half the cost of the same treatment at the hospital emergency room.

"WALK IN" MEDICAL CARE

When Kent Lemarie, MD, and Kenneth Gray, MD, co-owners of Emergency Medical Doctors, opened the center in 1981, there was only one other walk-in medical center in the San Diego area. Now there are approximately 20 (Lemarie and Gray now own two). In the United States there are more than 2,000 similar centers, which go by such names as emergi-centers, freestanding emergency centers, walk-in minor emergency centers, prompt care clinics, or urgent care clinics. And their numbers are growing. In one recent year some 12.3 million people were treated in these centers. It's predicted that before long there will be 28.8 million people using such facilities each year.

What exactly can a walk-in medical center do?

Dr. Lemarie explains the three major areas of emergency care. "First, there is the trauma victim—the automobile and motorcycle accidents. Next is the acute serious medical emergency—a heart attack, an out-of-control diabetic, or a person having seizures. We are prepared to handle these two groups—it would be unconscionable if we weren't. But the patient we have really geared our care to is the one with the episodic medical problem. This is the patient who can be given care in one or two visits. It could be the patient with a respiratory infection, or the one who steps on a rusty nail. Or it could be the high school athlete who needs a sports physical."

So no screaming ambulances will drop off critically ill patients at the Escondido facility. The walk-in center (and others like it), in fact, is run very much as a doctor's office—except it's better equipped than most doctors' offices and very modern in appearance.

Patients are first seen by a secretary-receptionist who gathers the usual information and discusses payment (which is cheaper than the same care at the emergency room and is usually covered by medical insurance). The patient is then escorted to the treatment area by a nurse who takes a brief history and may examine the patient. The physician then does an examination, makes the diagnosis, and prescribes treatment. Besides the physicians and nurses, there are technicians who take x-rays and run lab tests that assist in making a diagnosis. (In some walk-in centers there are also adjoining pharmacies that will fill prescriptions until late hours).

If a patient needs hospital care, he will first be stabilized at the center, then transported immediately to the hospital. Any patient who has a medical problem that requires more than one follow-up visit will be referred to a specialist.

This is how the ambulatory care concept works at the Emergency Medical Doctors Center. But there are no enforced standards for walk-in centers, and some may give less than adequate care. Some states have recommended that freestanding emergency centers (as well as ambulatory surgical centers) be subject to licensure standards designed to ensure the quality of care consumers receive.

All freestanding centers (minor emergency centers, ambulatory surgical centers, and birth centers) also can be certified by the Accreditation Association for Ambulatory Health Care (AAAHC). However, lack of accreditation does not necessarily reflect on the quality of care. At the present time certification is voluntary. Because it is costly and time-consuming, there are many well-run walk-in medical centers that haven't yet been certified.

Measuring the Quality of Care

So, how do you measure the quality of care? Barbara Saad, RN, nurse manager of the Emergency Medical Doctors Center, offers the following guidelines for determining quality.

Physical Setup—An ambulatory care center should have the equipment necessary to carry out most routine x-ray and laboratory tests. The facility should also be equipped with a "crash cart" (mobile emergency medicine chest), as well as a defibrillator, oxygen, monitors, and other lifesaving equipment. Most important, the staff should be qualified to use the equipment properly—specifically, physicians must be certified in advanced cardiac life support. Registered nurses should also have this certification.

Personnel—Ideally, owners of the facility should be licensed physicians who not only carry out administrative tasks but also examine and treat patients at the facility. Physicians should preferably be specialists in emergency medicine, family practice, or internal medicine. There should be a physician on the premises at all times.

There should also be an RN on staff at all times. The nurses should be experienced in emergency medicine. All office personnel should hold current CPR certification.

X-ray technologists should have state licensure and certification as a radiologic technologist by the ARRT—American Registry of Radiologic Technologists. At least the supervising technician—if not all the lab technicians—should have state licensure. Most important, unqualified office personnel should not be doing lab work, and aides should not be giving injections.

When walk-in centers first opened their doors, they had their share of critics. Some physicians called the quick-service establishments "Medical McDonald's" or "Docs-in-a-Box." Critics complained that one-stop medical care couldn't offer the emotional rapport that a patient can only obtain from a family doctor. And continuity of care would be broken if patients went from one walk-in facility to another. (In actual truth, up to 35 percent of adults don't have a family physician anyway.)

Many hospital emergency rooms, although threatened economically, thought the walk-in centers would go away. But the facilities seem to be here to stay, and many hospitals or medical plans have now decided to join 'em rather than fight 'em. Called urgent care clinics, these hospital-connected facilities offer longer hours for minor emergency problems. Their facilities are totally separate from the hospital emergency room but they have the advantage of hospital backup (if necessary) and greater continuity of care for patients.

A word of caution. Walk-in medical care is not for everyone. If you have a *serious* medical emergency, such as a head injury, you should go directly to a hospital emergency room. But if you have a minor medical problem, such as a suspected sprain or other injury, and you're traveling in a strange town, or are new to a community, or don't have a primary care physician, or your primary care physician is on vacation or otherwise unavailable, an ambulatory care center may be just what the doctor ordered. The walk-in centers are cheaper, faster, and more personalized than emergency rooms.

NEW PLACES
TO GO FOR DIAGNOSTIC TESTS

Twenty years ago, when Jane Moore was suffering from abdominal pain, she was hospitalized to have a few diagnostic tests done. First, there were a number of blood tests, then an x-ray examination of the gallbladder (using a radiopaque contrast medium). Finally, an upper GI series and a lower GI series were done several days apart. Mrs. Moore was in the hospital for over a week.

"The thing I remember most was that I was lonely and bored in the hospital. There was a lot of time between tests—a lot of time I spent stewing and fretting. I didn't really need to be in the hospital because I wasn't sick. But that was the way things were done then.

"The tests showed that I had a small duodenal ulcer. I took milk and antacids round the clock and took the medicine that the doctor ordered. The ulcer healed up just fine."

Now, at age 70, Mrs. Moore and her husband live in South Florida. Last year Mrs. Moore again suffered from abdominal pain. She went to her primary care physician and he recommended that she have a number of diagnostic tests.

"I had several blood tests in the doctor's office, then I had an upper and lower GI series done in our local diagnostic center. I went in on Monday for the upper—I was there a couple of hours—then the barium enema was done on Friday. It also took several hours, including the waiting time. But it was nothing really. My husband came with me both times. The rest of the week I went about my regular routine—puttering around the house, fixing my husband's meals. My life went on as usual, although I was a little tired on the afternoon I had the barium enema. The tests showed that I had a hiatal hernia and another very small ulcer. I understand that there's no real treatment for the hiatal hernia. With the ulcer, this time there was no milk and antacid round the clock—just antacid four times a day and these new pills that really did the trick."

When Mrs. Moore had to have the tests done, she went to a nearby freestanding radiologic (x-ray) center. It isn't connected to the hospital, and Mrs. Moore's physician refers all his patients there when x-rays are needed. Some diagnostic centers are also equipped to do blood work, take EKGs, and run even more sophisticated tests. There are also diagnostic centers that cater to women's needs only (mammography is provided along with instruction on breast self-examination). If the diagnostic center is well run, it provides an efficient and less stressful way to have tests done. It's also less costly and usually covered by insurance.

In communities where there are no freestanding diagnostic centers, tests can still be done on an outpatient basis through the hospital radiology or nuclear medicine departments. There are a few diagnostic tests that are more invasive and incur a certain amount of risk in themselves. They will require an overnight stay. The most common of these are arteriograms or angiograms; angiocardiograms or cardiac catheterizations; and myelograms.

If your physician has recommended one of the more risky tests, you should ask if there's a less invasive test that can give the same answer or can at least be tried first. If there is, have the test done at a diagnostic center or on an outpatient basis at the hospital. You'll be glad you did.

WALK-IN SURGERY

Johanne Glenn is in her 70s and lives in Boston. In 1982 she had a cataract extraction and a lens implant in her right eye. Johanne spent two nights at the local general hospital, as was the custom then. The cataract surgery went smoothly, but two years later a film formed over the new lens. In a ten-minute office procedure, this film was removed using a laser. One month later, Johanne Glenn had the same cataract extraction and lens implant surgery in her left eye. But this time the surgery was done at a freestanding eye surgery center, although the same ophthalmologist did all three procedures.

Mrs. Glenn compares her first surgical experience—as an inpatient—with the second when she was "in and out" in two hours.

"Both times I was satisfied with the care and the surgical result. But I recovered more quickly when I had the surgery done at the eye center. In the hospital I think they put me under a little more—it seems I was groggy for quite a while afterward and spent a long time in the recovery room.

"When I went to the eye center, I arrived at 10:30 in the morning. I had had my physical examination, lab work, and an EKG done at my regular doctor's office before the surgery. The eye doctor gave me a printed instruction sheet that explained the surgery and what I was expected to do—I got a similar sheet after surgery on what to do at home. Anyway, I was told what to wear on the day of surgery, and when I got to the eye center I just put a paper gown on over my clothes and put on a paper hat—it looked like a shower cap—and put paper coverings over my shoes. I didn't have to remove any clothing. During the operation, the doctor asked me questions and I was encouraged to talk (in the first surgery, I was not allowed to talk but told to remain as still as possible). After the surgery was over at the center, I had a turkey sandwich and orange juice—I was given a choice of several items for lunch. A nurse stayed with me during this time, took my blood pressure, and kept an eye on me. At 12:30 I walked out to the car and my husband drove me home. I didn't feel that anyone was rushing me to leave but I wanted to get home as soon as possible.

"In my after-care instructions I was told not to bend over and not to lift anything heavier than ten pounds for three weeks. My husband has had to put drops in my eye three to four times every day. But other than that, I've gone about my business as usual. When I went to see the doctor for my checkup, he commented that I was far ahead in my recovery from the surgery. As far as going to the outpatient center rather than going to the hospital, I would recommend it to anyone who's in good health—especially if their insurance will pay for it."

According to Mr. Glenn, the total cost of the surgery (including doctors' fees) at the hospital, in 1982, was $5,500. The total cost at the outpatient surgical center, in 1985, was $3,800. "Since we used the same surgeon both times, I can only assume that the center pocketed a portion—but a much smaller portion—of what would have gone to the hospital if Johanne had had the surgery done there again."

Mr. Glenn pauses for a moment and then comments, "I'll tell you the truth, if motels charged what hospitals do, nobody would ever travel!"

Of course, not all surgery can be done on an outpatient basis. Ambulatory surgery is meant for patients undergoing minor surgical procedures (a minor operation is one that does not require prolonged general anesthesia and extensive postoperative care). Ambulatory surgery also is not geared for the patient who is seriously ill or is a high operative risk because of high blood pressure, diabetes, heart disease, or other serious conditions.

In addition, some patients (particularly those who are elderly) may be nervous about the "in and out" aspect of ambulatory surgery. They may feel more comfortable staying overnight in a hospital "just in case something goes wrong" (all surgical centers should have hospital backup in the event that complications occur). Patients who live alone and are unable to get suitable help for the first day or two of convalescence may also be better off having surgery done in the hospital. One way of getting around the "in and out" apprehension of minor surgery is to get on the surgery schedule early in the morning. That way you can spend most of the day recuperating at the center.

It's currently estimated that 40 percent of surgery can be performed on an outpatient basis, and 50 percent of surgery will soon be done this way. At the present time, some of the more common surgical procedures done in ambulatory surgical centers are cataract surgery, tonsillectomy, breast biopsy, D&C (dilation and curettage of uterus), tubal ligation, vasectomy, some hernia repairs, knee arthroscopy and other minor orthopedic surgery, and face-lifts and other plastic surgery.

The Advantage of "In-Out" Surgery

Cost is probably the biggest reason why ambulatory surgery has become a popular alternative to inpatient surgery. The ambulatory centers can charge as little as one-third what a hospital charges. The reason is that, like walk-in medical centers, the surgical centers carry smaller overheads than hospitals because their facilities are less sophisticated. Additionally, hospitals frequently use the revenues from minor operations to help subsidize the more costly services, like open-heart surgery, whereas minor surgery is all that ambulatory centers do.

Insurance companies are now promoting outpatient rather than inpatient surgery whenever possible. Medicare has also encouraged wider use of surgical centers. Cataract extraction, the most common surgery for older people and the procedure that Johanne Glenn had, must now be done on an outpatient basis or Medicare will not pay.

For the patient who has no insurance, outpatient surgery is definitely the least expensive alternative.

Besides the cost advantage, there are other reasons why you should consider a surgical center. For the young mother who doesn't want to leave her family for several days or for the working person who doesn't want to miss additional days recuperating from surgery and a hospital stay, a surgical center can save valuable time. Additionally, if you're scheduled for surgery as a hospital patient, there's always a chance that your surgery will be "bumped," or postponed, one day if an emergency case arrives in the operating suite. This would never happen in an ambulatory center because only minor surgical procedures are done there.

Another important fact: Because ambulatory surgical patients are basically healthy and are in and out of a surgical center so quickly, there is less risk of postoperative infection.

The psychological advantages of ambulatory surgery are also noteworthy. Because the ancillary personnel in surgical centers work regular hours and only participate in minor surgery, they are under less stress than their hospital counterparts. What this means to the patient is a much more pleasant and personalized atmosphere. For the young child who needs minor surgery, this low-key approach can be one of the biggest reasons for having the procedure done in an outpatient setting. Having a parent constantly nearby and returning home to sleep in one's own bed makes minor surgery much less traumatic for youngsters.

Every person who chooses an ambulatory center feels less like a "patient" than the person who is admitted to the hospital. This can help speed recovery. For Johanne Glenn, feeling less like a patient meant being able to keep on her own clothes during the surgery. For another person it might mean being able to walk out of the center one hour after surgery and, with only a few restrictions, return to his or her normal life again.

TAKING YOUR BACK TO SCHOOL

Eighty percent of the population of this country has or will experience back pain. One-third of all worker's compensation claim costs are related to back pain and each year, over $14 billion are spent in legal costs, sick pay, and medical/surgical benefits for back injury and pain.

According to a recent Swedish study, the number of days lost to back injuries can be most effectively reduced through a program of education. In this study, researchers divided 200 low-back–injury workers into three groups. One group received physiotherapy, the second got a placebo (a "dummy pill" that has no therapeutic benefit), and the third went to back school to learn proper back care. The physiotherapy and school group both got over their symptoms in 15 days, about twice as fast as the placebo group. But the back-school students were back on the job in 20 days, compared with 26 for both the other groups.

The success of patient education for back problems has been demonstrated in this country, too. Liberty Mutual Insurance Company, for one, runs a back school in Boston where students learn proper back care.

Back schools instruct students in proper body mechanics for such activities as standing, sitting, lifting, reaching, and exercising. Students also learn ways to organize their environments for work efficiency and safety. The emphasis of the program is self-responsibility for a healthy back, 24 hours a day, at home and at work.

PAIN CENTERS

Henry Anderson, age 70, can pinpoint the moment his pain began. Sharp, severe sensations ravaged the inside of his head. Later, ugly lesions disfigured one side of his face. The cause of Anderson's disabling pain was a chronic form of shingles. The cure, however, was elusive. Anderson saw several doctors who prescribed acupuncture and a nerve-blocking injection. He also started taking regular doses of pain-killing drugs. Rather than help his pain, however, these only added to his misery and depression.

Like others who suffer from migraines, arthritis, back pain, pinched nerves, and other maladies, Anderson was beginning the terrible cycle of anxiety, depression, loss of appetite, profound fatigue, and sleeplessness. For 40 million people in the United States (one in six) and their families, chronic pain becomes a horrible way of life. And most physicians, trained to cure acute illness, are frustrated by patients whose pain refuses to go away. They frequently are unable to help.

Luckily, Anderson's physician referred his pain-wracked patient to the Scripps Memorial Hospital Pain Center in La Jolla,

California. One of 150 multidisciplinary pain clinics in the world, Scripps is primarily an inpatient program that treats individuals with chronic but nonmalignant pain. It has three phases. The first is evaluation and diagnosis of the pain problem. This is an in-depth work-up that often includes psychological, neurological, orthopedic, radiologic, and laboratory examinations as well as a thorough physical examination. If a physical problem is detected, the appropriate treatment is recommended.

In most cases of chronic pain, however, the cause of pain cannot be quickly fixed. What follows for patients admitted to the pain center, then, is a four- to five-week structured program that includes physical activity management (including daily exercise classes by a physical therapist), individual counseling with a primary nurse and group therapy with a psychiatrist, alternative pain treatments (including transcutaneous electrical nerve stimulation), and medication adjustment to decrease the dependency on drugs. In addition, there are discussions and lectures on the nature of the chronic pain syndrome, techniques to reduce pain, and education on drugs. Occupational therapy, biofeedback and stress reduction training, and family education and counseling are also provided. Weekly supervised outings practice pain control techniques in a social environment. Finally, when the inpatient period is over, there is an ongoing after-care program.

For Anderson, the program at Scripps was not at all what he expected. What he wanted to do when he began was rest in bed and comfort his pain. Instead, the staff kept him busy every minute. He was required to dress for breakfast, make his bed, attend vigorous physical conditioning classes, and interact with others in the program. After three weeks he was able to give up his dependence on pain killers and sleeping pills. This was a significant step. By the end of the program, his outlook on life was much improved. Although still not totally pain-free, Anderson has learned to live with his pain and take control of his life again.

Not all patients who enter the pain center are able to tell the success story that Anderson tells. Of those who enter the program, about 50 percent could be considered successful after six months. About 30 percent could be termed partially successful and 20 percent would have to be termed failures. However, that honest assessment of success/failure is much higher than any other option open to the patient whose life is consumed with pain. In addition, most of the patients who enter pain centers are at the end of their rope. They have sought relief from doctor after doctor and have suffered through numerous surgical procedures and years of drug dependency. Frequently, they have gone outside the medical system for herbal treatments, chiropractic care, faith healing, and other unorthodox methods.

Pain centers—whether offered as an inpatient or outpatient service—may not be the answer for everyone, but they're certainly a "safer" alternative than some traditional approaches for the relief of severe, chronic pain.

BIRTH CENTERS— A HOMEY ATMOSPHERE

"When I got pregnant the first time," explains Alicia Francis, "we lived in Atlanta. I knew from reading and talking to others what kind of birth experience I wanted, so I set about trying to find the right person to direct my care. I was interviewing obstetricians and went to one whose nurse told me to take off all my clothes so the doctor could examine me first. I did as I was told and sat their shivering in my paper drape until I suddenly realized it wasn't right. So I put my clothes back on. When the obstetrician came in the room, I told him I had put my clothes back on because I didn't know him and I wanted to talk first. Strangely enough, he understood perfectly and he became the doctor who delivered my baby—in a birth suite connected to the hospital. It was a natural birth and a very good experience.

"After we moved to San Diego and I became pregnant again, my husband and I again visited obstetricians. The ones we spoke with routinely used fetal monitors, IVs, and drugs and didn't hesitate to do a caesarean section. One doctor told us that 30 percent of his patients ended up having sections. I was appalled!

"When I was four and a half months pregnant, we were still looking for a doctor and also a hospital that had a philosophy similar to ours. We were getting discouraged. Finally we were referred to the San Diego Midwife Services, and it had everything we wanted. Janice Hutsell delivered our baby in the birth center. That was a year and a half ago and I still can't praise Janice and Roberta Frank (the other full-time certified nurse-midwife, or CNM) enough. They are extremely professional and knowledgeable, but the focus of the midwife's care is that the patient takes responsibility for herself whenever possible. That's very important to me."

Birth centers, which are usually staffed by certified nurse-midwives (experienced registered nurses with advanced degrees) are frequently referred to as obstetrical "halfway houses" because they provide the advantages of both home and hospital birth. Although there may not be a birth center in your community, the popularity of this alternative facility is increasing. It seems fitting, then, to look closely at one birth center where quality care is given by certified nurse-midwives.

A Day in the Life . . .

The San Diego Midwife Services opened for business in 1981, but since 1983 it has been housed in a one-story stucco building in an older residential area near Balboa Park. The facility is only five to seven minutes away from five major cooperating hospitals, and that fact is a comfort to the staff and their clients.

There are two entrances at the front of the building—one sign points to the office door, the other identifies the birth suite entrance. Entering the office side, one is impressed with the homey atmosphere that pervades this special place. There are several large collages of baby pictures hanging on the wall—satisfied customers all. On a side table there's a box of fresh fruits and vegetables with an invitation to "Take one." There are books and helpful pamphlets arranged in several parts of the room. Just around a corner there's an exchange box with baby and maternity clothes neatly stacked, just waiting for one of the clients to "help herself."

Carol, the office manager, has a large desk in one corner. She greets patients, answers the phone, and keeps track of who's coming and going. Beyond the waiting room is a hallway. Along one wall there's a large wooden examining table for babies. Five rooms open to the hallway. To the right is an examining room for gynecology patients—it has the usual examining table (albeit homemade), sink, and straight back chair. Down the hall is the prenatal examining room that houses a large bed for prenatal checks (this is in contrast to the usual uncomfortable examining table that obstetricians use). The prenatal examining room is large and is sometimes used as a second birth suite when the need arises. Also off the hallway there's a bathroom and a modest medical supply cabinet. (Nurse Hutsell explains, "We have the equipment to start IVs and do episiotomies, but frankly, the supplies aren't used often.") At the end of the hallway there's a small kitchen where patients and families can prepare meals and snacks. There's a full-sized refrigerator, sink, oven, and other equipment.

Finally, there's the birth suite, which looks very much like a regular bedroom with a large adjoining bathroom and a door that opens to the street. There are double windows along one wall of the birth suite that let in the morning sunlight. The double bed is covered with a blue velour comforter, which is removed when a patient is using the suite. There's a black-lacquered rocking chair and a nightstand in the room. A high-intensity stainless steel lamp stands in one corner—it's connected to a large battery unit in case of a power failure. The lamp is the only piece of stainless steel equipment that can be seen in the center. This is in contrast to the typical cold, shiny technological environment in which most babies are born.

Twenty-seven-year-old Linda Carr used the Midwife Services and explains her birth experience as, "the most exciting thing I've ever done. I'm especially glad I was able to do it my way."

The young mother explains: "When I first got pregnant, I knew there were certain routine hospital birthing procedures that I didn't want to have. I also liked the idea of a woman attending me rather than a man. Most important, I didn't want strangers around when I was in labor and delivering my baby. For these reasons I chose Midwife Services.

"As it turned out, there were four people in the birth room with me: my husband, a neighbor-friend, Roberta Frank (the CNM), and the RN who taught our prenatal classes. I felt very comfortable with each of these people, and everything went smoothly—my labor only lasted two hours! When I was in labor I chose a squatting position and found it so natural and comfortable that I delivered the baby that way. I would never have had that option in the hospital, where a mother lies flat on a delivery room table and pushes her baby out without the help of gravity. Also, I didn't want to have stitches, so the nurses used hot oil compresses on my perineum (the area between the anus and the vulva) to help stretch the tissues. There were no tears and no stitches.

"Several hours after the baby was born, he seemed to have some breathing problem and was grunting with each breath. The nurse-midwife immediately called the pediatrician at the hospital and he suggested bringing the baby in to be checked over. My husband and the RN took the baby to the hospital. It turned out that the baby was fine—he stayed at the hospital for a couple of hours and was put under a heat lamp. But the nurse-midwife didn't hesitate to seek additional help when she felt it was necessary. I liked that."

Total maternity costs at Midwife Services are about 30 to 60 percent of customary medical maternity expenses for the San Diego area (if hospital transfer is necessary, however, these savings may not be realized). Almost all insurance companies cover the care given at Midwife Services.

Janice Hutsell is quick to point out, however, that, "money should never be the determining factor in deciding on a birth center or home birth rather than the traditional obstetrician/hospital birth. I tell my clients they should first decide what they want in a birth experience, then decide on the provider."

If a woman decides to use the San Diego Midwife Services, the routine goes something like this: The initial one-hour consultation includes taking a history, doing a physical examination, and collecting specimens for laboratory tests. During pregnancy the patients are seen on the same schedule as with an obstetrician (every month up to the seventh month, every two weeks for two months, then every week until the baby is born). According to Nurse-Midwife Hutsell, visits with the CNM last at least 15 minutes, compared with the usual 2 to 5 minutes that is customary with obstetricians. She explains: "If patients can't think of questions to ask, we have a list that *we* feel they should be asking so we discuss those."

If at any time it is determined that the mother falls into a high-risk category (more about that later), then the patient is referred to an obstetrician who continues the care. If a home birth is planned, there are certain criteria that must be fulfilled and the home must be cleaned a special way. If the baby is to be born in the birth suite, the patient brings her own bed linen (to reduce the risk of infection), food, and other items.

When a pregnant woman thinks she's in labor, she calls the service switchboard and the RN on call checks the woman either at home or in the birth suite. Once it's been established that labor is in progress, the certified nurse-midwife is called. Nurse-midwife Hutsell explains: "I try to be there at the end of the first stage of labor. This transition time is when things start to get rough, and women may ask for pain medication. I find that my arrival is usually sufficient to 'do something' so that drugs aren't needed."

The CNM, the RN, and the support person (usually the father) all assist in delivery. Once it is born, the CNM examines the baby and stays until the infant is at least one hour old. The RN stays for two to six hours following delivery. The day after the baby is born, the RN visits the home. At two weeks and again at six weeks, baby and mother are seen in the office.

Nurse-Midwife Hutsell points out an important fact: "When babies are born, patients get five to ten times more care from a nurse-midwife than from an obstetrician. The doctor usually arrives at the end of second-stage labor, catches the baby, stitches up the episiotomy, and leaves. The CNM is often with the patient for five hours during labor, delivery, and after-care."

The National Picture

The National Association of Childbearing Centers is responsible for promoting the healthy growth of birth centers in this country. The organization works with a number of government agencies and private organizations to increase the number of centers and to educate the public in the advantages of this alternative birth style. The association also gives workshops on establishing centers and acts as a consultant for new centers.

According to this organization, there are presently 126 known birth centers in the United States. Although this number may seem small, the home-birth and birth-center movement has profoundly influenced birthing practices, leading many more couples to push for different approaches to birth. According to Nurse-Midwife Hutsell, rates of home birth have kept fairly stable, at 2 to 4 percent, since World War II. But she predicts that in 50 years or less, more than half the women in this country who do not select home birth will deliver their babies in birth centers. As one new mother put it, "We women have done this—we've created a real revolution in how we want our babies to be born."

But Is a Birth Center for Everyone?

Prospective parents who choose either hospital, birth center, or home birth will find studies to substantiate that each is safe and that each is potentially dangerous. So the decision of where your baby should be born is, to some extent, a matter of style and personal preference.

But there are some expectant mothers who should never consider having a baby outside of a hospital setting. These are the high-risk mothers and they usually fall into one of the categories listed below:

WOMEN NOT SUITABLE FOR DELIVERY AT HOME OR BIRTH CENTER

- First mothers who are over 35 years of age; any mother over 37 years of age.
- Any acute or chronic medical problem in the mother, including anemia, diabetes mellitus, heart disease, or kidney disease.
- Complication in previous pregnancy—including caesarean section.
- Rh incompatibility.
- History of very large or very small infants.
- Small pelvis in mother.
- More than four previous deliveries.
- Problems during present pregnancy such as pretoxemia or toxemia, abnormal presentation, or bleeding.

Even if a pregnant woman has none of the listed "complications," she may still opt for a hospital birth if she feels emotionally more secure being in a fully equipped facility with highly trained obstetricians only minutes away (the low-risk mother should consider, however, that these obstetricians may *cause* more problems than they solve).

There is also a certain group of women who have a low threshold for pain and absolutely insist on "something being done" when the pain of labor becomes intense. Obviously these are not women who would be good candidates for delivery at home or in a birth center. Regardless of where a woman has her baby, the presence of a caring, supportive person is a real asset in reducing pain and speeding up labor.

If a low-risk expectant mother wants the security of being in a hospital but also wants the relaxed style practiced by nurse-midwives, she might consider a hospital birthing suite.

New Innovations in Hospital Births

Hospital policies vary considerably in what is allowed for an alternative birth experience. Some hospitals—especially those located in areas where home births are popular—are willing to let doctors and nurse-midwives perform the kind of low-key delivery that might be done at home or in a birth center. Some allow families, including siblings, to stay together the entire time. Others have simply redecorated one room to look like a birth center but continue to operate by the same rules that are so objectionable to some parents. In some hospitals, in fact, birth rooms are there strictly for decoration. Very few women get to use them because their doctors insist that "the mother's condition warranted more conventional care."

If you want to make sure that you have the most natural experience possible in a hospital setting, you should ask the following questions (before the time of delivery): How many women actually use the birthing room and how many are turned away because of "complications"? How many women require labor-inducing drugs, fetal monitoring, and caesarean sections? What "standard obstetrical procedures" (like enemas, shaving of the pubic area, use of IVs) can be eliminated? Who is allowed to stay with the mother during labor and delivery?

As a prospective parent, you want to do the right thing. If having your baby at home or in a birth center sounds like the best alternative, make certain that the provider is either an obstetrician in good standing or a certified nurse-midwife (very few physicians now attend home births because of the fear of malpractice suits; however, some do deliver babies in birthing suites adjacent to their offices). Besides the obstetrician or nurse-midwife, there should be at least one other trained assistant at the birth. Preferably this should be an experienced RN. The health provider that you select should offer adequate prenatal care and classes. A nurse-midwife should follow strict, conventional guidelines for transferring care to an obstetrician and/or hospital. Finally, the home or birth center that's selected should be only minutes away from a cooperating hospital that can provide care for both mother and baby.

Most important, is the basic philosophy of the health provider similar to yours? Are your concerns and desires taken into consideration and do you feel comfortable with the person you've selected to supervise your care?

Giving birth should be one of life's happiest and most triumphant moments. The choice of how and where your baby will be born is a personal decision that deserves careful thought and investigation.

THE RIGHT TO DIE IN PEACE

A dying patient is the one that hospitals handle least well. To the medical staff the dying patient is seen as a failure—so even when the patient has reached the point of letting go, the medical staff will order one more x-ray, do one more treatment, or perform one last heroic gesture (such as CPR) "just in case." To the nursing staff the dying patient is a symbol of the mortality that everyone tries to avoid. Because it's so painful to face, death is kept in the back room, eyes are averted, the patient and family are left alone to cope and to grieve as best they can.

At the turn of the century 70 to 80 percent of Americans died at home. Today it's just the opposite—80 percent die in hospitals and nursing homes.

But dying patients have an alternative to the impersonal and technological world of today's hospital. They can select a hospice program and experience a more peaceful and comfortable end to life.

What Is Hospice?

Hospice is both the oldest and the newest concept in providing care for the terminally ill. The word "hospice" stems from the Latin for "host" or "guest," and it was originally a medieval haven for weary European travelers, a place for replenishment, refreshment, and care. The modern hospice was inspired by St. Christopher's, which was established in 1967 in London. In Britain hospices receive funds from the government and are widely used.

The first hospice in this country was the New Haven Hospice—a home care program founded in 1973 by Sylvia Lack, MD, who trained at St. Christopher's.

In the United States nine out of ten hospice patients have cancer. Usually the patients are elderly and all have less than six months to live. Besides caring for cancer patients, hospice programs can also serve people who have limited life expectancy because of kidney, heart, lung, and neuromuscular diseases.

In this country hospice can mean a program, a type of care, or a facility for the terminally ill and their families. Wherever hospice care is provided, the goals are similar:

- Ease the pain and treat the symptoms of patients who have a short time to live (usually six months or less).
- Enable patients to spend as much of their time as possible at home in familiar surroundings, with patient and family members still in control.
- Help the patient's family cope with the illness, subsequent death, and bereavement process.

Most hospice programs require that the patient's own physician direct the care. However, hospices use a team approach to meet the complex physical and emotional needs of dying patients and their families. It is not unusual to find a physician, nurse, home health aide, social worker, pharmacist, clergyman, psychologist, and other workers actively involved in a patient's care. Volunteer participation—by both professionals and nonprofessionals—is considered to be part of this team approach.

The difference in cost is substantial. At-home hospice care is a fraction of the cost of traditional hospital care, while a stay in a hospice unit is about two-thirds the cost of a hospital stay. The actual cost to an individual patient will vary depending on the patient's diagnosis, insurance plan (or Medicare eligibility), and the individual hospice. The personal warmth of hospice care and the absence of "heroic" measures cannot be put into dollars and cents, but these features are undoubtedly the most important reasons for choosing this alternative.

The hospice movement in this country has been a movement toward care of the terminally ill patient at home. There are various ways to organize hospice care, and programs differ from community to community (to find out if there's a hospice program near you, write to the National Hospice Organization, 1759 Old Meadow Road, McLean, VA 22102).

One way to find out about hospice programs is to see one in action. Let's take a look.

A Visit to One Hospice

One of the few inpatient hospice units in Southern California is run by a health maintenance organization, Kaiser Permanente. This 17-bed facility is located in Norwalk just off Highway 605—one of Los Angeles's busiest freeways. The Kaiser hospice program has proved very successful, and as of this writing there are plans to establish two more hospice programs in the Los Angeles area, as well as one in San Diego and another in Northern California. The Kaiser facility has demonstrated its popularity with patients and administrators. How did the project come about?

In July 1978, Kaiser started a hospice home care program with money from a National Cancer Institute (NCI) grant and Kaiser funds. In January 1979, the inpatient hospice opened its doors.

The inpatient facility is nestled within a larger complex of Kaiser offices and another inpatient unit. It's immediately apparent, however, that the hospice section is a very different place.

Patients and visitors enter through a landscaped courtyard and open the front doors to a large family room. There's a fully equipped kitchen on one side of this room and a large parlor on the other. The parlor is attractively decorated and houses a large television set and a cage of chirping parakeets (a gift from a former patient). Patients and visitors are free to use the family room facilities any time of the day or night.

Patients' rooms are located on either side of the family room and form a "U" shape around the courtyard. In this way, each of the eight two-bed rooms (and one single unit) open to the outdoors by sliding glass doors. In nice weather, patients can be wheeled to a small patio area in the courtyard—there's also a park one block away where patients can visit.

The rooms are modern and cheerful and some have been personalized with pictures and belongings from home. Cots can be put in rooms if family members want to spend the night (a special room is also available for visitors who live out of town and want to stay with a dying relative for a longer period of time).

There are some other unique areas in this hospice. The chapel room is open 24 hours a day for patients and visitors, and has been the setting for a number of weddings and funerals. The stained-glass window depicts a western outdoor scene and was donated by a grateful family member. Next to the chapel is the viewing room, which resembles an ordinary bedroom. After a patient dies, the body is placed on the large bed and friends and relatives are encouraged to come to the room and say their final good-bys. Across the hall from the viewing room is a children's playroom, which is used by visiting youngsters. It is also in this room where Ozma Mantele, a staff nurse with additional training in child psychology, does play therapy and sand play with the children of dying patients. Mantele works with those youngsters who are experiencing loss and grief and helps them to express their emotions freely.

Mantele is but one of the members of the hospice team at the Kaiser facility. George Espe, MD, a specialist in internal medicine, has been with the program since it started in 1978. Richard Brumley, MD, a specialist in family practice, joined the staff in December 1981. There are also two full-time social workers, a full-time volunteer director, and a chaplain who works with patients and staff members. The nursing staff (registered nurses, licensed vocational nurses, and aides) work on a flexible schedule that is determined by patient census. Staff nurses wear no uniforms.

Dr. Brumley, who works in both the home care and inpatient units, explains, "I'm frequently asked how I can work in a hospice. Believe me, it's not that grim a place. People are honest about things here—patients know they have cancer and there's no sneaking around about that. The staff is very open with their feelings too. We had a 39-year-old patient, for example, who was terminally ill with breast cancer. She and her husband were celebrating their 15th wedding anniversary, and the patient had written a beautiful poem for her husband. We have a music therapist who works for us part time. She put the patient's words to music, taped the song, then presented the tape to the patient and her husband as an anniversary gift. I can tell you that the whole staff was crying that day. And that's not the only time we've been moved to tears."

Because of the strong support among staff members, there's low staff turnover at the Kaiser hospice. Many of the nurses have been with the unit since it opened in 1979. Dr. Brumley describes one problem he initially experienced: "When I first joined the hospice program, it was hard for me to get out of the old mold of treating all medical problems aggressively. In hospice we look first at what patients and families want."

What *do* cancer patients who are terminally ill usually want? In Brumley's view, "Most patients want to be home in quiet, familiar surroundings." Even though only 35 to 40 percent of the Kaiser patients die at home, they receive most of their care, until the time of death, through the home care program. The usual census of hospice patients is 10 to 12 inpatients and 40 to 45 home care patients.

To qualify for the hospice home care program, the patient must be a member of the Kaiser HMO and live within a 25- to 30-mile radius of the Norwalk facility. The patient must have been seen by an oncologist (a specialist in cancer treatment) and have a diagnosis of cancer (the three most common cancers treated in the Kaiser hospice are lung, GI tract, and breast cancers). When surgery, chemotherapy, or radiation therapy can no longer increase life or when the patient refuses additional therapy, it's time to turn to hospice care, where quality of life rather than cure becomes the goal.

There are five full-time RNs in the home care program—two are public health nurses. There's also one full-time home health aide. Other nursing personnel are called in as the need arises.

When a terminally ill cancer patient is referred to the hospice program, a registered nurse from the staff visits the home and meets with the patient and family. An important criteria for home care is that a relative or friend can take responsibility for the patient's care and be available 24 hours a day.

On the first home visit the nurse discusses the hospice program, answers questions, and obtains informed consent from the patient (or a family member) to participate in the program. In hospice, patients are aware of their diagnosis and prognosis. Since a cure is no longer possible, the issues become pain control and physical comfort as well as emotional and spiritual support. No one is forced to become a part of the hospice program, and in fact, according to Dr. Brumley, "There are a small number of patients who say they are not ready for hospice, or we occasionally meet family members who change their minds and want the patient treated more aggressively. That's their choice and we always abide by their wishes. Hospice is a valuable option, but it's not right for everybody."

Once the patient has been accepted into the program, a team, including a physician, nurse, social worker, and perhaps a home health aide or volunteers, is assigned to the patient.

Either Dr. Espe or Dr. Brumley makes an initial assessment visit, then visits the patient periodically. The home care nurse visits about twice a week to provide care, keeps a check on symptoms, and shows the family how to provide for the care and comfort of the patient. A hospice nurse who knows about the patient's care is available 24 hours a day by calling the hospice telephone number.

Kaiser provides all home equipment, including hospital beds, oxygen tanks, bedside commodes, suction machines, or whatever is needed. Drug coverage varies with the patient's health plan but is the only item for which the family would have to pay. For Kaiser the cost per home visit is $93, while the cost of one day in the hospice facility is $234 (both of these figures exclude administration costs and physicians' fees).

A patient in the home care program is admitted to the hospice facility when symptoms—such as pain, nausea, or constipation—get out of control. If the patient is admitted, he or she may stay from eight hours to several days or until the problem is resolved. Other patients from the home care program are admitted to the facility for up to a week for respite care. This time is given to family members who need a break from the demands of providing care. There's another category for which patients can be admitted to the hospice facility. This is the patient who has a life expectancy of less than two months and is not able to be in the home program (usually because the patient lives alone and has no one who can be responsible for care). In the past such a patient would have been admitted to a nursing home to die. The hospice is seen as a more humane alternative.

Fifteen-year-old Yvonne is an unusual patient at the Kaiser hospice. First, she's young (the average age of patients in the hospice program is 62). Second, she has suffered from a malignant brain tumor since age three but, until recently, was responding well to standard therapy. Yvonne knows, however, that the doctors can do no more for her and that she will soon die. Yvonne's cancer is spreading rapidly, and at the time of admission she is blind and is beginning to lose her hearing.

Yvonne is one of five children in her family, but since age three she has required the greatest amount of help and support from her parents. The lives of her siblings have been greatly affected by their sister's illness. To provide her parents and siblings with some rest and some time to sort out their own lives, Yvonne has been admitted to the inpatient facility. It is in this place, too, that the ailing youngster plans to spend her final days, preferring to die there rather than at home.

Yvonne is small for her age and her frail body is almost swallowed up by the adult-sized hospital bed. The 15-year-old is a charming youngster with large brown eyes and a ready smile. She quickly catches the hearts of the staff members as they provide supportive care and help Yvonne and her family to express their feelings and emotions during these difficult last days. Elaine Quillian, the social worker assigned to Yvonne's care, is planning an "unbirthday party" for the youngster. It is to be held several days later in the hospice family room. A guest list is made up, games and special music are planned. Nothing is left to chance—Yvonne even gets to pick the color of the roses on her cake. There will undoubtedly be laughter and tears at the unbirthday celebration—it will probably be the last event that the teenager can enjoy.

After Yvonne dies, her family will continue to receive help and support through the hospice bereavement program. They will be counseled by the social worker, chaplain, or a psychologist—as needed—and will be encouraged to join a number of support groups. The same volunteers who assisted during Yvonne's final days will also stay in touch during the time of bereavement. The hospice staff will try in every way they can to help Yvonne's family during the time when their lives will be so heavy with grief.

Elizabeth Hospice—Home Health Agency

The Elizabeth Hospice of Escondido, California, was started in 1979 by four RNs (three of whom were named Elizabeth). Betty Bulen, one of the original founders, is the present executive director. Elizabeth Hospice began as a community, or volunteer-based, service program. In 1982 it became licensed as a home health agency. The program is funded by local contributions, grants, and third-party payments, and is available 24 hours a day, seven days a week. It is a member of the National Hospice Organization.

As of 1985, Elizabeth Hospice has provided ongoing care to 1,000 patients plus family members. When one considers that this community-based operation has less than ten paid staff members, the level of service is very impressive. It's volunteers—neighbors helping neighbors—who get the job done. Two hundred and fifty strong, the volunteers are the backbone of Elizabeth Hospice. They work in the office, run a thrift shop, and do other jobs as needed. Seventy-five serve as patient care volunteers, and the human support and understanding that these workers provide is the key to the success of this organization.

One volunteer explained her minimum four-hour-per-week "job": "I feel that the greatest service I give as a patient care volunteer is emotional support to the terminally ill patient and his family. That can mean sitting at the bedside and offering a comforting hand to the dying patient. Many times patients have told me that it means so much to them for me to be there—to be in touch and caring. Then there's the support that we give to family members. That can be time spent listening or it can mean contacting family members or making funeral arrangements when that becomes necessary.

"As volunteers, we frequently do grocery shopping, run errands, take patients to the doctor's office, or stay with patients so that family members can be free for a while. Sometimes we help by taking a family member out to lunch or for a ride. In one situation, the patient I was helping was paralyzed and needed to be turned every two hours round the clock. The patient's husband was doing this alone and was exhausted. So for two nights a week, I stayed at the house and turned the patient. On another night, one of the other volunteers spent the night. That gave the husband three nights a week when he could get his rest. This went on for three months. Another time the patient died when I was at the house and his wife asked me to stay. I never left her side for three days. I arranged for the minister and family members to come and stayed until the patient was cremated, and even went out on the boat with the widow when the ashes were strewn at sea.

"I feel rewarded that I can do these things for people. The little things I do make their lives somewhat easier during the stressful period of terminal illness."

Who becomes a patient care volunteer is determined by a mutual screening process, although the hospice staff ultimately determines if the prospective volunteer will be able to do the intense and difficult work that is required. Patient care volunteers must attend a 36-hour training program that includes learning simple physical care techniques for seriously ill patients and developing communication skills.

At Elizabeth Hospice there is a three-hour patient care conference twice a month. The first hour and a half is spent with a physician, a clergyman, representatives from other community organizations as needed, members of the hospice staff, and the patient care volunteers. All aspects of the patient's care are discussed. The second hour and a half is spent with just the volunteers and patient care coordinator. The volunteers are encouraged to share their own emotional needs, and the staff provides a supportive and safe atmosphere in which to do this.

The use of volunteers in Elizabeth Hospice embodies the spirit of friends helping friends—neighbors helping neighbors. This fact contributes to the tremendous success and growth of this organization. The use of volunteers also builds a strong community support system and is cost effective. For these reasons Congress has determined that Medicare reimbursement for hospice care will be given only if volunteers are a part of the hospice program.

Hospital-Based Hospice

As has been pointed out, a hospital is probably the worst place for dying patients. A home care program or a freestanding hospice unit puts the greatest distance between the patient and technology, and this is an advantage to the dying patient. Placing a hospice program in a hospital setting tries to put the proverbial square peg in a round hole.

But hospice is not so much a facility as it is a philosophy of care for the terminally ill. A few hospitals have set up hospice units that are treated as separate entities, and the units work closely with effective home and volunteer programs. One shining example of an effective hospital-based hospice program is the one at Mercy Hospital in Rockville Center, Long Island (this facility was used as a model in the National League for Nursing book *Hospice—The Nursing Perspective,* edited by Sylvia Schraff, RN, MSN).

Some nursing homes are also making a greater effort to respond to the special needs of the dying patient. But it's an uphill struggle for many.

Guidelines for Determining Quality of Hospice Care

In some communities, hospital or nursing home hospices are all that's available. To assist you in deciding if a hospice program measures up, you should ask the following questions:

- What is the program's philosophy on heroic measures? For example, does the staff administer CPR or use lifesaving equipment for the dying patient? They shouldn't.
- What is the program's philosophy on pain control? There should be definite medical guidelines for prescribing pain

medications, and the staff's goal should be to provide maximum safe pain relief to patients.

- Do hospice workers work exclusively with the hospice program or do they "float" from one job to another? Because hospice is so different, the best workers are those who have specialized in the field.
- Is the patient's dignity and autonomy recognized and respected by the staff? Will the patient's religious beliefs (or lack of them) be respected?
- Does the hospice have a physician or RN on call 24 hours a day, seven days a week? If you have a primary care physician, what will his relationship be with the hospice staff?
- Does the hospice have a strong volunteer program? Does the hospice offer a bereavement program? These are both essential ingredients to effective hospice care.
- How much of the hospice service is covered by insurance, and what services, if any, are provided free of charge?

Chapter 6

HOSPITAL ALTERNATIVES YOU SHOULD AVOID

It's been estimated that Americans spend more than $10 billion every year on worthless and often dangerous treatments. That's a lot of money for nothing more than shattered dreams and disappointment!

Some who chase such rainbows do so because they are disillusioned with the present medical establishment and would prefer to be more active participants in their health care (there's a great amount of validity in the new trend toward self-care, but if carried to extreme, it can be dangerous). Some who choose unorthodox healers do so because these providers *seem* to understand their clients' emotional needs best and they usually promise quick (but quacky) magical cures. Still others patronize health hustlers out of desperation.

I don't want you to be one of them.

So, let's discuss some of the more notorious treatments that should be avoided. By knowing the risks involved and promises claimed in such so-called treatments, you'll be able to make a wiser decision should the time come for you to make a choice.

LAETRILE CLINICS

Jack White, 55, was at the end of his rope. Diagnosed as having inoperable lung cancer, he underwent limited radiation therapy and was told by the cancer specialists that his chances of living longer than a year were doubtful.

A good friend told Jack about the miracles of Laetrile therapy, and after talking it over with his wife, Jack decided to seek treatment at a clinic in Tijuana.

At the Mexican clinic Jack was impressed with the clean and professional appearance of the building. Everyone seemed friendly and concerned. The young Mexican doctor, who was in charge, spoke English fluently. He wore a white lab coat, had a shiny stethoscope tucked in his pocket, and looked very professional. He answered all of Jack's questions and told of one clinic success story after another. The doctor was sure he could help Jack, and Jack was willing to let him try. After all, what did he have to lose? Having been written off by the cancer specialists, Jack White now had hope that he could be cured. So he admitted himself to the clinic for one month of Laetrile and nutritional therapy.

Jack was not a foolish person but he was desperate. The warm and understanding attitude at the Mexican clinic was a far cry from the cold, technological atmosphere of the American hospital where he had initially been treated. At the Mexican clinic he felt more like he had some power over his treatment. He could ask questions and have them answered. Sometimes he wasn't sure what the Mexican doctor was talking about, but many times he hadn't been sure what the American specialists had been talking about either.

After one month of inpatient care, Jack returned home with a three-month supply of Laetrile stashed in his suitcase. After he was home for a month, a strange thing happened. Jack felt better. His appetite improved, he put on weight, and he and his wife did some traveling. But after a year he had a relapse and the Mexican clinic could no longer help him. He died in an American hospital. It was 18 months after the original diagnosis had been made.

Since 1920, Laetrile—an apricot-pit extract—has been described as a cancer remedy first by the California father-and-son team of Ernest Krebs Sr. and Jr. and then by a host of followers. In spite of the drug's popularity, there is no valid scientific evidence that Laetrile works in curing cancer. Not only does it not work, but cyanide poisoning is a side effect that can occur with the administration of Laetrile. So why do so many cancer victims opt for this form of treatment?

The case of Jack White could not be classified as a cure. But his life *was* extended six months beyond what the cancer specialists predicted, and he enjoyed several pleasant months. Why? His family credited the Laetrile therapy but probably the limited success was a result of two phenomena: the "placebo effect" of the Laetrile and the temporary remission that White experienced either naturally or as a result of the radiation therapy.

First, the placebo effect. From the moment he walked into the clinic, White anticipated that he would get well and all the clinic personnel reinforced this. Regardless of whether the Laetrile had any genuine effect in relieving symptoms, White believed that it was beneficial and so it was. Call it the power of suggestion or faith or hope, it was something that White and almost all cancer patients *need.* It is a failure of traditional medicine that many physicians don't provide this hopeful, positive attitude that is so necessary to recovery.

Second, the phenomenon of temporary remission. Cancer is a disease that is characterized by temporary remissions or periods when symptoms improve. White's use of Laetrile probably coincided with a natural remission, although Laetrile got the credit. It also could be that the temporary remission was due to the radiation therapy that White received in the American hospital.

Jack White spent a good deal of money and put his faith in medical quackery. He did it because he was desperate. The will to live and avoid suffering is strong in all of us. Jack was no different. He grabbed for the nearest lifeline and believed the unbelievable promises.

Some might say, "So what's the problem? Every patient should have the right to pick the treatment of his or her choice. White hurt no one when he was taking Laetrile. And he only took the drug after traditional medicine gave up on him."

True enough. But what of the next cancer patient who could be saved by conventional treatment but instead opts for the worthless Laetrile? And what about the hucksters themselves—the con artists who prey on innocent victims? If even a hopeless patient patronizes a quack, this helps to keep the business alive and reinforces the charlatan's reputation.

CHELATION THERAPY CLINICS

Elderly patients suffering from heart disease, arteriosclerosis, or other illnesses associated with aging go to the clinics once a week for therapy. They sit in recliner chairs and receive intravenous medicine or chelation therapy from one of approximately a thousand doctors or clinics in the country who offer it. Most of the elderly patients swear by the treatment.

The process of chelation, which uses a man-made amino acid (EDTA), is believed to work by bonding the amino acid with heavy metals, such as calcium, copper, iron, and lead, in the body. According to its advocates, this allows excess metals in the body to be excreted through the kidneys. Its proponents say that chelation can eliminate the need for 75 percent of all coronary bypass surgery. And the therapy has been advertised as a cure for blindness, senility, Parkinson's disease, muscular dystrophy, and other diseases.

In 1953 the FDA approved chelation for treating lead poisoning. But in 1983 the federal agency said that other unapproved medical purposes for using the therapy (such as for treatment of arteriosclerosis) constituted mislabeling.

Detractors have called chelation "quackery practiced by licensed physicians," and insurance companies have refused to reimburse patients for such therapy. In May 1983, an American Medical Association panel of experts found chelation to be an "unacceptable or indeterminate" therapy for arteriosclerosis. And all the experts agreed that it had potential dangers. Some of these dangers were decreased levels of ionized calcium that could lead to irregular heartbeats, convulsions and respiratory arrest, depression of bone marrow function, and kidney failure.

And yet, from New York to California, elderly people believe in the treatment and they keep going every week for chelation therapy.

ARTHRITIS "CURES"

There are no cures for most kinds of arthritis. There are treatments that can bring remission and relief from pain. But no cures.

People don't want to have a chronic painful disease like arthritis and they probably don't want to be told that they must be an active participant in an imperfect treatment program. Arthritis sufferers don't like to hear these words, so many turn to practitioners who never mention such things and promise a simple, easy, and exclusive cure. And any remedy, no matter how controversial or bizarre, can seem inviting to an arthritic who is in pain.

Because the symptoms of arthritis come and go, people often connect improvement with an offbeat treatment rather than a natural remission. When patients tell their friends about the amulet or potion that did the trick, a "cure" is born and another health hustler enjoys fame and fortune.

Because 35 million to 40 million Americans suffer from arthritis, the promoters have a huge market to draw from. For some patients, using unorthodox remedies only results in a waste of money or a loss of dignity (they find they have been duped). For other patients, however, the consequences are more serious—the side effects are even worse than the disease.

What are some of the magical "cures" that have been offered to arthritis sufferers over the years.?

- Smearing the body with cow manure "mud packs."
- Sitting for prolonged periods in an abandoned mine in Utah, Colorado, Wyoming, or Montana to absorb the healing radiation or drink or bathe in the radioactive waters found in the mines.
- Undergoing a series of "flu shots."
- Taking pills derived from the yucca plant.
- Ingesting liver juice and cod liver oil (to "lubricate the joints").
- Following starvation diets.
- Receiving injections for bee-venom desensitization.

A number of these worthless arthritis "cures" have faded from the marketplace and we may laugh at them now.

But what about wearing a copper bracelet or using a vibrating device to cure arthritis? Or what about hormonal compounds (combinations of cortisone and male and female sex hormones) that cost at least $500 for a six-month supply and can be purchased in Mexico, the Dominican Republic, and a few U.S. "clinics"? None of these measures is an effective treatment for arthritis.

The bracelet and the vibrator will probably not harm you (the copper bracelet especially seems to offer a placebo effect for many), but the large dosages of hormones can cause thinning of the bones, lowered resistance to infection, high blood pressure, cataracts, glaucoma, peptic ulcer, and diabetes. Would anyone really want to trade these conditions for a momentary lessening of arthritis pain?

One treatment that never seems to go away is the use of colonic irrigations for the treatment of arthritis (it's also used as treatment for skin problems, gallstones, and cancer). A hose is inserted into the rectum and water is run through all six feet of the colon. It is not an effective treatment for arthritis and can result in a ruptured colon or an infection from using either a contaminated hose or contaminated fluid.

Then there's treatment with cobra venom, various vitamin therapies, soaking in mineral or sulphur baths, and swallowing concoctions made from alfalfa seeds or watermelon seeds. The list is endless.

The truth is that there is no one simple cure for arthritis because there are many different forms of the disease—some mild, some severe. But for the millions who suffer from arthritis, there are many orthodox treatments—including medication, rest, and exercise—that are effective.

When it comes to arthritis "cures," then, it's in your best interests to duck the quacks and consult a physician who practices standard diagnostic and treatment procedures.

OTHER UNCONVENTIONAL "HEALERS"

- Five-year-old Shawn Henry developed leukemia and was being treated at the local children's hospital. While Shawn's parents watched in horror, their son suffered through chemotherapy and radiation treatments. It seemed to Shawn's parents that the treatment was worse than the disease, so they went to a "metabolic therapist" who counseled them (for a sizable fee) and gave the boy massive doses of vitamin A (at a cost of more than $100 a month). Fortunately for Shawn, he also continued his treatment at the hospital. Some months later, Shawn's leukemia was in remission but he was terribly ill from vitamin-A poisoning. He complained of severe headaches, dizziness, and excruciating bone pain. X-rays revealed the damage that the vitamin A had done—there were bone abnormalities and swelling of the boy's brain. Ironically, Shawn almost died—not from the leukemia but from the megadoses of a fat-soluble vitamin. Shawn's parents are suing the "metabolic therapist."

- Eighteen-year-old Doris Barber was trying, again, to lose weight. This time she had consulted an herbalist who recommended drinking large amounts of a preparation containing tonka beans, wood-ruff, and melilot. She also took large amounts of vitamin A, and because she suffered from headaches, took aspirin regularly. As a result of taking this combination of drugs, Doris experienced abnormal menstrual bleeding and other problems. Her blood's clotting ability had been reduced because of the drugs. It took a number of anxious months before Doris was herself again.

The snake oil peddler is alive and well in this country. He no longer drives a horse and buggy or gives his pitch at the local carnival. These days he peddles his wares in television commercials and through flashy ads in newspapers and magazines. The products promise to remove wrinkles, cure baldness, develop a woman's breasts, reduce weight effortlessly, cure impotency immediately, or offer you a shiny machine that can rid you of every disease known to man. All these pills, tonics, and gadgets can be ordered in the privacy of your home (enclose check or money order). But will they work? The chances are: never.

No one wants to be duped and no one wants to throw away money. So, as a rule of thumb, it's best to have any medical problem investigated first by a licensed medical professional and at least try the conventional treatment before considering any alternative care. And then before starting treatment with an unconventional health provider, do some research on your own in the medical section of your local or university library. Has the unconventional provider demonstrated documented effectiveness in his area of expertise? Articles supporting the proposed therapy should be published in professional journals and be based on documented research rather than just testimonials. Does the "doctor" have an MD degree? Has the person been licensed to perform the treatment in question?

Another source of information is a trusted doctor. Ask him about the proposed treatment or contact the appropriate voluntary agency, such as the Arthritis Foundation, the American Cancer Society, or the American Heart Association.

Be skeptical if any medication promises to cure a number of unrelated ailments. No one drug can be all things to all diseases. And don't assume that medications cannot be sold without FDA approval. Products can be sold for a number of years before the FDA can take action. And by the time that happens, the hucksters have left town and are on to their next scheme.

Treatments by practitioners of chiropractic and acupuncture are now considered by many in the medical community to be relatively safe alternatives to conventional medicine (although they once were not acceptable). Many of these less conventional practitioners are trying to move into the mainstream of traditional medicine and they're very aware of their limitations.

But there are other practitioners who feel they have no limitations. These healers use strange titles after their names like ND (doctor of naturopathy), PhN (philosopher of naturopathy), or MsD (doctor of metaphysics). These practitioners have no legitimate credentials and can only back up their health claims with testimonials or letters rather than with legitimate research. These would-be healers promise quick miraculous cures, and that's what every suffering patient wants to have. But if there were such a dramatic breakthrough, wouldn't you imagine that the medical community would be pleased to hear about it rather than have the secret kept under a basket? And if the cure were legitimate, don't you think that members of the business community would be banging on the healer's door to have a piece of the action?

The quack frequently claims that he's being persecuted or is misunderstood by other doctors. This could very well be true. The persecution is for good reason. Quacks share their secrets with the vulnerable and take their victims in. They prey on the sick and promise the impossible. No one needs these slippery folks, but like death and taxes, they'll always be with us.

So it's the health consumer who must be wary—it's the consumer who has the power to make or break the charlatan's claims. Be skeptical—don't be taken in by the impossible cure.

Chapter 7

THERE'S NO PLACE LIKE HOME

Eighty-three-year-old Louisa Guillio, although terminally ill with cancer, has chosen to cope with her illness at home rather than in a hospital or nursing home. Angie, her retarded daughter, is in her late 50s and has always lived with her mother. Neither woman is yet ready to break their long-standing relationship, although they know, because of Mrs. Guillio's illness, that death within the next several months will separate them forever. For the present, however, Louisa can move around in her familiar four-room Denver apartment and Angie can provide some small comforts for her.

It is mid-March—a pleasant sunny day that hovers between winter and spring. Louisa sits in her favorite chair in the living room amid possessions and souvenirs collected over a lifetime. In one corner, a tall glass cabinet displays several shelves of framed family photographs. There are knickknacks and pictures neatly arranged throughout the apartment. Louisa's daughter Angie sits at the kitchen table finishing lunch. Her chair is situated so that she can watch her mother's every move.

Joan Cooper, RN, is visiting Mrs. Guillio. The nurse is part of a growing number of health care professionals who provide services to the sick and disabled in their homes. Nurse Cooper wears a white lab coat over her regular clothes and sits on a stool next to Louisa. She holds the older woman's hand and speaks in a calm and soothing voice.

Mrs. Guillio is talking about her relationship with her daughter Angie."If I didn't have her, I don't know what I'd do. Just gettin' me things—bringin' me a glass of water—it's a help. And it's nice to have her company."

Hearing these words, Angie hides her head in her hands, then sits up and beams with pride. "I do the best I can do, Ma."

Louisa is quiet for a moment then suddenly clutches her stomach and cries out, "It's that gas. . ."

Nurse Cooper walks to a side table, "I'll get your medicine."

The white-haired patient, her face distorted in pain, takes the spoonful of antacid offered by the nurse. "I've got to get up—I've got to help myself."

Nurse Cooper helps Louisa to her feet, then supports her patient as they walk slowly around the apartment together, finally returning to the chair. The pain is relieved but the anxiety remains. The nurse speaks gently, "Can you breathe with me, Louisa? Take it in and let it out slowly."

Following the nurse's directions, Louisa begins to relax. Daughter Angie, still watching from the kitchen table, also breathes with the nurse and relaxes. It's a brief moment of peace and tranquility— a moment to be savored.

Nurse Cooper has known the Guillio family for almost a year. Home health care was necessary following Louisa's surgery for colon cancer. The doctors later determined that the cancer had spread to her lungs. Louisa was recently seen by a radiologist who noted that the tumor in the lung was growing and that the prognosis was very poor. No further medical treatment was recommended.

In the beginning, Nurse Cooper visited Mrs. Guillio every day. There were daily injections for pain, dressing changes, and counseling on nutrition and health care. At first, care was aimed at rehabilitating the patient and returning her to a normal life. Now that it's been determined that Louisa's illness is terminal, care is aimed at increasing physical comfort and providing emotional support.

Nurse Cooper has recently cut visits back from five days a week to three. Care is supplemented with visits from a home health aide on the other two days. Mrs. Guillio's younger daughter, Jan, who lives in town but is married and has a family, will begin to take over more of her mother's care. She has also agreed to have Angie live with her after Mrs. Guillio dies.

On this March day, the biggest priority in Mrs. Guillio's health care is pain relief. In recent months, a number of drugs have been prescribed by the family physician but they were either ineffective or caused significant side effects. Mrs. Guillio is now taking methadone by mouth every three to four hours round the clock (methadone is a synthetic narcotic pain reliever with actions similar to morphine). Nurse Cooper has instructed her patient to write down the time that she takes the medication, and this log is shown to the nurse each time she visits. To relieve the nausea that is a side effect of methadone therapy, Nurse Cooper puts a circular patch behind Louisa's ear. This patch, which is impregnated with scopolamine, is changed every three days by the nurse. In the patient's opinion (the opinion that counts the most), the patch is most effective in "settling my stomach."

Another priority in Mrs. Guillio's care is providing adequate nutrition. Because of nausea and gas pains (partly a side effect of methadone therapy, partly a result of the cancer), Louisa's appetite is poor. She is sometimes afraid to eat because of "choking feelings" and fears of "food getting stuck." But she knows she must eat to keep up her strength, although sometimes a meal is only a few sips and a couple of bites. Nurse Cooper usually plans her visits around breakfast time (with a follow-up telephone call in the afternoon). The home health aide prepares supper on the days that she visits. On weekends, Louisa's daughter Jan does the marketing and helps in food preparation. Mrs. Guillio could have the services of Meals on Wheels for a minimum fee. They would provide a hot noon meal and a bag supper five days a week. Mrs. Guillio decided against the service preferring to "do for myself"—and enjoy her favorite ethnic dishes—for as long as possible. Mrs. Guillio is absolutely opposed to tube feedings or intravenous therapy, and her wishes will be respected by those who supervise her care.

Unlike the situation in a hospital or nursing home, patients in home health care programs can determine when and what they want to eat. They can also gauge their level of activity to their biological clock rather than to the hospital clock.

Mrs. Guillio tires easily and decides to lie down in her bed for a while. While she rests, Nurse Cooper calls Mrs. Guillio's daughter Jan and discusses the patient's condition. The possibility of inpatient hospice care has been discussed on a number of occasions, but

Mrs. Guillio has decided against it. Nurse Cooper answers Jan's questions about the patient's decreased appetite and her general condition.

The home nurse then contacts the home health aide who will be visiting the next afternoon. Besides preparing the evening meal, the aide will give Louisa a bath, a shampoo, and a back massage to help her relax. As Nurse Cooper explains, "Providing comfort is the main objective now."

After the brief rest, Nurse Cooper examines Louisa and checks her blood pressure, heart rate, and other vital functions. She tells the patient her findings—nothing is held back—and tells her that the doctor will be ordering oxygen to help relieve her shortness of breath and anxiety. Louisa isn't happy that oxygen will be necessary—it's another reminder that her body is failing her. She decides to forgo it for the time being.

Louisa sits on the edge of the bed and grips the mattress to give her support. She seems to have found new energy and talks candidly about her situation.

"This [home health care] is a good thing. People want to stay home—it's the best. My doctor can't help me now. Nurses spend more time with you anyway—they're more understanding. Having Joan [the home health nurse] has been wonderful. I've known her so long. She's like my daughter. As long as I can call her, I'm not afraid to die here. Here in my own bed—not in some strange hospital bed."

Before leaving, Nurse Cooper spends a moment with Angie, who suffers when her mother is having a "bad day."

Nurse Cooper drapes her arm around Angie's shoulder and listens sympathetically. She understands Angie's situation, and the two talk about this new life that's been thrust on the family. The months ahead will be even more difficult for Louisa and her daughters. A great amount of physical and emotional support will be needed. This long-term, in-depth relationship is both an advantage and a challenge for providers of home health care.

THE MANY
FACES OF HOME HEALTH CARE

Home health care for Louisa Guillio and her family is provided by Partners Home Health, a proprietary (profit-making) agency. But similar services could also be provided by the Visiting Nurse Association (VNA), the local health department, a private nonprofit agency, or a hospital-based agency. Proprietary and private, nonprofit agencies are the newest providers in the industry and, combined with the others, are making home care increasingly available for Americans.

But who are the providers and how do they meet the needs of their clients? How is it affordable? Let's take a look.

The Visiting Nurse Association

The VNA is the oldest type of home care agency and is particularly strong in the New England states. VNAs offer skilled care through large, well-established agencies and provide most of the home care in this country. (Visiting nurses, who see many patients, should not be confused with private-duty nurses, who give more extended care to one patient at a time.) Service is given to any person who needs health care, regardless of ability to pay. Because payment is made on a sliding scale, VNAs frequently have clients who pay no fees. For this reason, agencies often have to depend on fund-raising or donations from such charitable organizations as the United Way and Easter Seals. VNAs offer a wide variety of services and generally charge less per visit than other agencies.

Government Agencies
or Public Health Departments

Although these providers have the largest number of Medicare-certified agencies, they do not see the largest number of clients and are expected to cut back even more as time goes by. Like VNAs, health departments have a policy of treating any patient in need, regardless of ability to pay. Funding for government agencies depends on the budget of the particular city, county, or state.

Hospital or
Nursing Home-Based Agencies

These facilities are seen as extensions of hospitals or nursing homes and receive referrals through the provider organization. According to figures from the Health Care Financing Administration, institution-based agencies that are Medicare certified fall below the norm in terms of the number of visits per patient, although they are much higher in average charge per visit and average charge per patient.

Proprietary
(Profit-making) Agencies

Privately owned and profit oriented, these agencies are the fastest-growing segment of the home health care industry. Many of the larger health chains, such as Upjohn Health Care Services, Medical Personnel Pool, and Staff Builders, are proprietary agencies. Proprietaries are growing at a rapid rate because, since 1980, they can be certified and can provide services to Medicare beneficiaries in all states. In addition, these agencies offer a wide range of services (including, in many cases, supplying private-duty nurses and live-in companions to assist in home care), which are available 24 hours a day. Because of sophisticated marketing techniques, the public has become more aware of what these agencies offer.

Private, Nonprofit Agencies

These tax-exempt agencies are usually owned and managed by individuals or families. Although the agencies are generally small and offer a more limited variety of services, they see a large number of clients—particularly those covered by Medicare. Like the proprietary agencies, the private, nonprofit facilities are usually more expensive than a VNA or government agency.

Taking Care of Costs

The most recent figures from the Health Care Financing Administration on comparative costs per visit and per patient at various types of Medicare home health agencies appear on page 99.

But don't let any of these figures alarm you. Even for those who *can* afford it, payment doesn't necessarily have to come right out of your pocket. There are plenty of ways to cover the cost of home health care.

	Government	VNA	Hospital Based	Proprietary	Private Nonprofit
Average cost per visit	$ 26	$ 29	$ 38	$ 38	$ 39
Average cost per patient	$543	$647	$809	$981	$1,109

Medicare—This federal insurance program for the elderly and disabled was established in 1965, and in addition to other benefits, provides for health care in the home.

There are two sections to Medicare. Part A benefits are automatically provided to all eligible persons and include hospitalization, limited nursing-home care, and home health care. Under Part A, reimbursement for services and supplies is based on 100 percent of reasonable cost.

Part B provides supplementary insurance for medical services and is available to those elderly persons who enroll and pay a monthly premium. Part B usually pays 80 percent of the reasonable cost of such services as doctor's care, home health care, some therapy services, and laboratory and diagnostic services, as well as ambulance fees and cost of durable medical equipment and medical supplies.

Home health care is covered under both parts of Medicare and there is no limit on the number of visits. To be reimbursed for services, it is no longer required that a patient show previous hospitalization, but it is necessary to have a physician's order for care. To take advantage of Medicare's benefits, the patient must be homebound and in need of skilled nursing services or physical, speech, or occupational therapy on a part-time, intermittent basis. All services must be furnished through a Medicare-certified home health agency. At the beginning of this decade only 3.4 percent of Medicare enrollees used home health services. Hopefully, as the quality of home health care becomes more appreciated, more Medicare enrollees will take greater advantage of it.

Medicaid—A joint federal/state program, Medicaid assists low-income families and individuals finance their medical services. There are federal regulations that list the minimal services each state must provide. Home health care is included in this list, but the level of coverage and eligibility requirements vary significantly from state to state.

It's been estimated that Americans spend $30 billion a year putting people in nursing homes. About half of this amount is paid for by Medicaid. A much cheaper and more humane alternative would be to spend more money for health care and supportive services in the home and thus keep patients in familiar surroundings for a longer time.

Title XX of the Social Security Act—This program supplies social services for both the elderly and low-income families. It is supported by both federal and state funds and has as one of its major goals the prevention or reduction of inappropriate institutional care by providing community-based or home-based care. Along these lines, states have set up day care centers for adults, homemaker services, chore services, and home management assistance. The last three of these services may be offered by home health agencies in addition to their usual nursing and therapy programs.

Private Insurance—Most Blue Cross and Blue Shield policies include home health care in their coverage. This insurance plan generally offers such benefits if it will shorten or eliminate the need for a stay in a nursing home or hospital. Home health care is available only if a physician is in charge of the patient's treatment program. With Blue Cross and Blue Shield there is usually a co-payment feature, in the most common of which the patient pays 20 percent of the cost. Generally, costs are covered only for recovery from an illness, operation, or nonchronic disability.

Other insurance plans vary in their coverage of home health services and medical supplies and equipment.

Other Sources—Home health services can also be paid for by the Veterans Administration, Champus, worker's compensation, federally qualified health maintenance organizations, and some social service agencies. For information on eligibility and coverage, contact the specific agency.

Self-Payment—Because VNAs and government agencies have a sliding scale for home visit charges, services may be free, minimal, or full price depending on your ability to pay.

Many proprietary agencies actively solicit patients who do not depend on third-party payments and can afford to pay out of pocket. For the proprietary agency, this means less paperwork, and money is usually received more quickly. For the patient, using such a proprietary agency may mean a greater array of services, but it also may mean a higher bill.

A LITTLE HISTORY

Home health care. There's nothing revolutionary about the concept. The first home nurse was probably a woman who dragged her mate from the field of battle to the warmth and security of a cave. This first home nurse probably wrapped her patient's wounds with strips of animal skin and cooled his feverish brow with damp compresses. She may have administered herbal medicines, prepared certain foods, and cared for her "patient"—as needed—until he was strong enough to do battle again (or until he met a peaceful death).

In colonial America, women were nurses to their families and neighbors. If home remedies failed, a doctor was called. Only the very poor or homeless went to hospitals. As organized medical and hospital care developed, home care was still seen as a viable alternative although there were no formal agencies or specific programs for the sick-at-home.

In 1885 the first nongovernmental, nonprofit agency specifically organized to provide home nursing care was established in Buffalo, New York. Other such agencies, later to become visiting nurse associations, opened offices in Boston and Philadelphia in 1886. In 1898 the Los Angeles County Health Department became the first official health department to provide home nursing care to the sick poor. In these early years the nurse's function was to provide limited physical care as well as to teach cleanliness and nursing skills to the patient and his family.

Until the late 1940s the VNAs and government agencies were the most popular providers of home health care (a few private insurance companies also offered limited home nursing care to policyholders, but their impact was small). Until 20 years ago, VNAs were solely dependent on donations and fees to finance their activities; government agencies were supported solely by tax dollars.

Beginning in the late 1940s, some hospitals were getting into the home care business. It seemed a natural extension of hospital service—referrals could be easily obtained and comprehensive care could be provided by those existing hospital staff members who specialized in the fields of rehabilitation, social service, or nutrition. A special home nursing department could be formed or nurses could be hired on a contract basis (usually working with an established Visiting Nurse Association). Patients could also be seen easily by physicians and referred to x-ray and laboratory units as needed. However, since private insurance companies were not committed to health care given outside hospital walls—and did not reimburse for such services—there was little incentive for institutions to expand home care programs.

Twenty years ago, when Medicare, Medicaid, and private insurers began reimbursing for home health care, things began to change. Proprietary agencies and private, nonprofit agencies are now competing with the traditional VNA, government, and hospital-based agencies for a bigger share of the home health care business.

Ten years ago half a million people received home health care; the figure has grown to two million today. In some parts of the country expansion has been at a phenomenal rate. In a one-year period, for example, Dallas, Texas, experienced a threefold increase in agencies, from 28 to more than 75. The National Association for Home Care estimates that there are about 5,000 home health agencies, 5,000 homemaker-home health aide agencies, and 1,200 hospices in the United States.

The presence of so many different home health care agencies can be cause for confusion. For the individual patient home care can be a blessing or it can be a disaster. Much depends not only on the patient's medical condition but also on his or her social and economic situation. Would home care be for *you*?

POSITIVES OF HOME HEALTH CARE

The most important advantage for those who choose home care is that the quality of life for patient and family is improved at home. Since the family, rather than the hospital, is in control, the patient can maintain a normal routine, have care adapted to his or her needs, or even reject care if desired. The home schedule does not have to be rigid or arbitrary but can be adjusted to the patient's wishes. The importance of eating off familiar dishes, dressing in one's own clothes, and sleeping in a familiar bed can only be appreciated after one has been stripped of these privileges in a hospital or nursing home.

When a patient is cared for at home, the usual support systems—family, neighbors, friends—remain intact. Besides giving a patient a sense of security, it places responsibility for patient care with loved ones and reinforces family bonds. Home care allows patients to relax and be themselves. It also encourages independence, which can help speed recovery. Additionally, health education of the patient and family is better accepted in the home rather than in the artificial and transient atmosphere of the hospital. Finally, the at-home patient avoids many of the usual hospital risks, such as infection, poor nutrition, and any of the other hazards I described in chapter 1.

Recently the American Association of Retired Persons surveyed its members and found that the vast majority—no less than 80 percent—would prefer long-term home health care to a long-term nursing-home stay.

Home health care sounds like the perfect solution for patients and their families. But . . .

THE PITFALLS
OF HOME HEALTH CARE

For some families home health care—as it is now set up in this country—is not feasible. Unless a family is wealthy enough to pay for the continual (round-the-clock) services of a professional nurse and a home health aide, much of the job of caregiver will fall to a family member (usually the spouse). If a patient's care is very complex or the patient is incontinent (unable to control bladder and bowel functions), home care may be out of the question. If the caregiver is in poor health or is physically small and frail (and/or the patient is large and heavy), attempting home care may result in two patients instead of one.

Also, if it appears that care will be long term and physically demanding, some family members may feel that they don't have the physical or emotional resources or the time to provide needed care. In today's society many women have carved out careers for themselves and they are not about to return to home and hearth and carry out the demanding tasks that are required of the main caregiver.

THE HOME HEALTH CARE TEAM

Physician—This is usually the patient's primary care physician and is considered the captain of the team. Specifically, the physician outlines and periodically reviews the patient's program of care in the home.

What kind of physician is best for home care? Internists and general or family practitioners are usually those best qualified. The home care physician should be available for occasional home visits and should be willing to supply phone numbers in case of emergency. You should be able to talk easily with the home care physician about medical and nonmedical problems, and he should be willing to work with health care agencies and refer you to other sources if necessary.

Nurse—The nurse provides the most service in any home care agency and is the professional the patient sees most often. Registered nurses (RNs) supervise the home care program and provide complex care. Licensed practical nurses (LPNs) and licensed vocational nurses (LVNs) sometimes provide more routine care to patients under the supervision of an RN. The services of an RN cost more than those of an LPN or LVN.

Public health nurses (PHNs) are RNs with additional education (minimum baccalaureate degree) in the field of public health. The PHN often works in a health department setting and coordinates services to improve the health and well-being of the community. The PHN may also coordinate services in a Visiting Nurse Association or proprietary agency.

A visiting nurse is an RN, but not necessarily a public health nurse. The emphasis for the visiting nurse is on the individual patient rather than on the community at large.

Some patients are all but impossible to care for—their personality may be difficult or they may be emotionally disturbed. If a marriage has never been strong or has been constantly filled with conflict, and the main caregiver will be the spouse, it may be best for all concerned to consider institutionalization (unless another family member can assume responsibility for care). Also, the home care patient may suffer if the family is embarrassed by the patient's condition and limits his or her social contacts.

A significant obstacle to providing home care is the facilities that are available in a community. In New York City and other large cities, many health agencies have the capability of providing very complex care for their clients. Administering chemotherapy in the home, for example, is not second best to providing this sophisticated

Private-duty nurses, though often working in the home, are not usually considered to be part of the agency home health care team.

Home Health Aide—After the professional nurse, this worker provides the greatest amount of service in home care. Aides provide personal care and supportive services under the supervision of a nurse. Training is usually short (six weeks to three months) for home health aides. These personnel are not licensed or certified by any national organization but are supervised by the employing agency.

Medical Social Worker—When part of the home care team, this person provides counseling, and finds and coordinates resources in the community.

Registered Dietician or Nutritionist—Frequently hired as a consultant, this professional plans special diets and assists patients and other personnel in managing nutritional problems.

Rehabilitation Therapists—Physical therapists, occupational therapists, and speech therapists are important workers in almost every home health agency.

Respiratory Therapist—As more seriously ill patients with respiratory problems are cared for at home, this therapist will become an even more visible member of the team. Respiratory therapists help patients with breathing problems. Their goal is to restore lung function or maintain function at its highest possible level.

Volunteers—Whether offering telephone reassurance, friendly visits, or transportation assistance, these unpaid workers are becoming increasingly more important in many agencies.

treatment in the hospital—home care is probably the *best* alternative for many patients. But if a cancer patient lives in an isolated area of the country where home care services are not as comprehensive, providing "high tech" treatments at home may be out of the question—a hospital stay will be necessary. In some areas even rehabilitative services are not adequate to meet the needs of the community. In such cases care in a rehabilitation section of a general hospital is the best alternative.

Some communities may have adequate medical programs for the homebound, but such services as transportation, meals, and housekeeping services are not sufficient or are too expensive. Not all agencies combine health services with chores and personal care, but for the vast majority of the elderly and chronically ill, the availability of these domestic services is the most important factor in keeping patients home rather than having them institutionalized.

To provide effective home health care, family members will need support from the medical community. They should live within driving distance of a hospital where the patient can be taken in case of emergency.

Then there's the matter of medical supervision. If the family physician is opposed to the idea of home health care, suggesting that it will be unsafe for the patient and/or devastating to the family, it's unlikely that the family will succeed with this approach (what the physician may really be saying, of course, is that he doesn't want to be inconvenienced by house calls or doesn't want to deal with community agencies that he sees as a threat to his authority and his livelihood). For whatever reason the physician discourages a family's efforts, it's best to discharge that physician and find one who will support the family and supervise the patient's care.

AND STILL
MORE SUPPORTIVE SERVICES

As I mentioned before, perhaps the biggest pitfall of home health care is that the burden of care and responsibility falls on the family. While she can make it possible for a person to be cared for at home rather than in the hospital, the visiting nurse or public health nurse only spends a relatively short period of time in the home— about an hour per visit. And part of the time is spent showing the patient and the caretaker how *they* can perform certain skills and carry out the physicians's orders. But for those who can afford it there is a way to relieve much of this burden. You can hire a nurse.

Private-Duty Nurses

Unlike a visiting nurse or public health nurse, private-duty nurses assume total care for a patient. Rather than an hour a day, they put in an eight-hour shift. They will follow the physician's orders, and if necessary, will feed, bathe, and provide whatever procedures and comforts are necessary.

If the caregiver is frail or works or is otherwise unable to give such nursing care, a private-duty nurse can be a valuable asset. Additionally, as the trend to earlier hospital discharge continues, some families may find that the services of a private-duty nurse are essential. However, their services tend to be expensive (by calling around in the San Diego area, I found that the usual hourly charge for a private-duty nurse was $20 to $30 per hour for an RN and $15 to $20 per hour for an LPN/LVN. Medicare does not cover this service and insurance plans vary in what they pay.)

If your insurance plan does cover the services of a private-duty nurse in the home, or if you can afford such a service out of pocket, what is the best way to find a competent nurse?

Many proprietary home care agencies have private-duty nurses on staff. Nurses' registries and employment agencies also refer and place such personnel in the home. You can find out whom to call by looking in the Yellow Pages of the telephone book under "Nurses and Nurses' Registries" or "Nursing Services." A better way to obtain the services of a competent private-duty nurse is to ask the opinion of an RN who is employed by a VNA or a government agency. These nurses would presumably have no financial ties to profit-making agencies or registries, and since they work in the field every day, they would have valid opinions on who's "good" or "not good." When inquiring about the cost of private-duty nurses, remember that an RN charges more than an LPN/LVN and a home health aide charges the least of all. These three levels of worker would not provide the same service, however, and some insurance companies will only pay for a private-duty nurse who's an RN—not an LPN/LVN. In addition, some agencies set a minimum number of hours a day or days per week for service. So even though these agencies would charge less per hour, the actual cost per week would be more because they require a minimum amount of service.

Home Management Services

Some critics of the present home care system stress that the area of home management is the one that the government has ignored. These critics argue that if an elderly, chronically ill person could have more assistance with meal preparation, marketing, housecleaning, and performing other household chores, there would be less need for institutional care. At the present time, government programs only pay for such assistance on a short-term basis (if at all). And private insurance is practically nonexistent for this kind of help.

For the average patient, assistance with household chores comes from family and friends. For those who are alone, there are a few social programs that provide household services, but many of the elderly are forced to either ignore the usual domestic amenities or reach into their pockets and hire help from private housecleaning or homemaker agencies. On a regular basis this can be quite expensive.

If a patient is receiving health care through a home health care agency, it's best to discuss the need for household help with that agency. Each community differs in what it's able to offer patients—a visiting nurse should be able to advise clients on what is available.

Meals on Wheels

For a small fee the elderly homebound can receive a hot noon meal and a bag supper delivered to their door. Food is usually prepared at such community locations as schools, churches, or senior centers and is available Monday through Friday. To qualify for the service, a person must be elderly and confined to the home. For further information on this very popular service, contact the local Meals on Wheels in your community.

Transportation

How does a homebound patient get out for doctor's appointments, medical tests, or just socializing with friends? In some communities it's a real problem. Many senior citizen centers run minibuses or vans and charge a nominal fee for rides. Other social agencies, churches, or hospitals may also provide this service—often there's no charge. The American Cancer Society has a Free Wheeler program in many communities. To receive free rides to and from treatment centers, a patient must have a diagnosis of cancer and must be ambulatory. There are no age or financial limits.

Reaching Out for Help

AT&T has devised an Emergency Call System-Medical Alert that links the elderly, the handicapped, and those with chronic health problems to one of two preset user-programmed emergency numbers. Several other companies offer similar help to the homebound. How do these systems work?

The AT&T system consists of a console and a portable transmitter. The console hooks up to any modular telephone jack and 110-volt outlet. The transmitter is designed to be carried conveniently in the hand or around the neck on a cord. In the event of an emergency, the user simply presses the button on the transmitter and the console automatically dials the first of two preset, user-programmed emergency numbers (this could be the fire department, paramedics, or the local hospital). It then gives all the pertinent information, by electronically synthesized voice, to the party who answers the call. If there is no acknowledgment from the first number, the system will automatically dial the second number. If the message is not acknowledged, the cycle is repeated. When confirmation is received, the console announces "message received" to let the user know that help is on the way.

AT&T has set up a toll-free number that consumers may call to get the name of the dealer nearest to them. The number is 1-800-431-1000; in Nebraska, 1-800-642-8300.

Adult Day Care

Most communities have a senior citizens center that provides meals and supervised activities at regular times. These services, however, are limited to those elderly who are in good health. For the older person who is handicapped, many states have opened day care centers that provide needed health services and are staffed by nurses, physical therapists, and nutritionists. Participants usually spend two or three days a week (from 10 A.M. to 3 P.M.) at these centers, receive health supervision, participate in an exercise and social program, and receive a nourishing meal. The remainder of their time is spent at home.

Adult Foster Care

This option allows elderly adults to live with families willing to share their homes. For certain elderly people this is a more humane and inexpensive alternative than the use of a convalescent home or a live-in nurse.

This type of program, which was started in 1982 by St. Francis Hospital in Poughkeepsie, New York, inspired a Lubbock, Texas, nurse named Jeanette Vaughan to start her own proprietary business called Senior Foster Services. Most of the foster families she has selected are divorced or widowed women or older couples. The families receive training in an intensive five-day class that emphasizes home health-aid skills, CPR, nutrition, and communication skills. Foster families are visited once a week by Nurse Vaughan to make sure they are providing the agreed-upon care.

The elderly clients or their families pay a fee to the service, which in turn pays the foster-care families. A foster family receives $500 a month for each client, regular days off, and one week's paid vacation during their first year of service (Vaughan compares her fee with the usual $1,200 a month charged by convalescent homes and live-in nurses).

Four types of foster care are offered: full-time service, short-term care immediately following hospitalization, interim care for those needing help between visits, and eight-hour day care. The program does not handle people with major health problems.

According to Nurse Vaughan, "Foster-care services will be an increasingly more popular alternative to hospital and nursing-home care. There are already 25 such programs in the nation (mostly in the Northeast), and interest in the concept is growing. Because it's a more personal type of service, foster care encourages emotional growth and physical independence."

A variation of foster-care programs that a number of communities are experimenting with is *shared living arrangements*. In this type of program, homeowners aged 55 and older are screened and matched with other people over 55 who are in reasonably good health but are in need of affordable living quarters.

Some communities have *independent living centers,* which are cooperative housing for the handicapped. *Halfway houses* are another alternative that permit the moderately disabled to live in a homelike atmosphere that provides companionship and supervision.

For more information on alternative housing for the elderly and the handicapped, consult the social service department of your local hospital, home health agency, or health department.

Adult Protective Services

This agency provides legal and financial counseling to those unable to manage alone.

DETERMINING
THE QUALITY OF CARE

Home health care should help relieve a patient's and family's physical and emotional burdens—not add more worries with unexpected costs or unsatisfactory performance. One way to avoid the unexpected is to investigate agencies before selecting one. The following criteria will help in this process.

Reputation and Care

What is the professional reputation of the agency? Is your physician familiar with its practices? How long has the agency been serving the community? You can contact the local chamber of commerce or Better Business Bureau to get one measure of the agency's reputation. Talk with other patients and families who used the services of the agency. Were they satisfied?

How does the agency provide care? A nurse or therapist should conduct an initial evaluation of your needs in the home. This should include consultations with the family physician, family members, and other health professionals. There should be a written plan of care. This plan should include what duties are to be performed and by whom. The plan should state at what intervals service will be given and what is the expected duration of care. The family should be allowed (and encouraged) to undertake as much of the care as possible. The professional who supervises the care plan should visit the home regularly. If questions or problems arise, these should be cleared up in a reasonable period of time. You should see most of the same faces week after week—continuity of care is important for you and the health worker. Ideally, nurses should be available for consultations and emergency visits 24 hours a day, seven days a week.

The Financial Picture

You should know, right from the start, how much home care will cost. Ideally, you should receive a written statement regarding financial arrangements. You should know whom to pay, when you will be billed, when payment is due, and if there will be any extra charges for certain services.

Home care is usually paid for in a number of ways. A reputable home health agency should be willing to work with all third-party payers and to discuss your financial situation at any time.

Check for Credentials

Is the agency licensed, bonded, certified, or accredited? What do these words mean?

Licensing is a basic legal requirement that all agencies must have in order to operate. Usually an agency is licensed by the state health department. The agency should be licensed, although this will tell you very little about the quality of care that is offered.

An agency and/or its employees also can be bonded. This is a protection for the agency in the event of a lawsuit but does not assure clients that quality care is provided.

The fact that an agency is Medicare certified is another measure of quality. To be certified, the agency must have met certain minimum requirements in financial management and patient care. Even if your care will not be paid for by Medicare, it's best to choose an agency that's approved by Medicare.

Accreditation is a voluntary process, and many agencies have yet to undergo the necessary work involved. It does not mean, therefore, that if an agency is not accredited, it doesn't measure up.

It is felt by many health care workers, however, that the process of accreditation would protect the health consumer at a time when a large and varied number of home health agencies are entering the market. Eventually accreditation will be a significant criterion for the consumer in selecting a home health agency. A number of nonprofit professional organizations provide accrediting services. These are: the Joint Commission on Accreditation of Hospitals (JCAH), which accredits home care services that are a part of a hospital program; the National League for Nursing (NLN) and the American Public Health Association (APHA), which jointly accredit freestanding home health agencies and community nursing services such as visiting nurse associations; and the National Home Caring Council (NHCC), which accredits programs that provide home-maker–home health services.

To receive a list of those agencies that have successfully completed the NLN accreditation process, write to the National League for Nursing, Division of Accreditation Services, 10 Columbus Circle, New York, NY 10019-1350.

TURNING YOUR HOME INTO A HOSPITAL

Even for those families who are committed to the *idea* of home health care, the *reality* of providing such care can seem very formidable.

Where does one begin? How can someone who is uneasy about illness possibly be a home nurse? And what about equipment and learning all the necessary skills? While the following section cannot replace a home nursing course, it might ease some anxiety for patients and caregivers as they sail into unfamiliar waters.

Selecting the Sickroom

During a brief illness there is usually no need to plan a special room for the sick person, and regular bedroom furniture will do very well. But with a long illness it is necessary to provide space where the patient will be comfortable, and where the home nurse can look after the patient as conveniently as possible.

If you live in a two-story house, it would be best to have the sickroom on the first floor, adjacent to a bathroom and fairly near the kitchen. In some families—especially those with no young children living at home—the family room, living room, or dining room is the ideal location for the sickroom. Such an arrangement is convenient for the caregiver, and being in the mainstream of family life may be more beneficial to the patient than being isolated in a bedroom. Every patient and every family situation is different, however. Some patients would prefer the privacy of their own room during evening hours but would enjoy a change of scene (the living room couch or easy chair) during at least part of the day. The sickroom should provide a delicate balance between a quiet and restful haven and one that does not promote boredom and isolation.

Regardless of where the sickroom is, it should have a large window that provides ventilation, lets the sunshine in, and allows the patient to feel a part of the outside world. Being able to watch the comings and goings of neighbors and to observe the change of seasons helps to contribute to a sense of normalcy for the homebound sick person. The importance of "feeling normal" should never be underestimated.

In selecting and setting up the sickroom, it often helps to have a visiting nurse from the hospital or home health agency come to the house and offer suggestions. Ideally this should be done before the patient returns home from the hospital or as early in the home care period as possible. The nurse's main concerns will probably be comfort, efficiency, and safety. Selecting the sickroom, rearranging furniture, removing scatter rugs, deciding which equipment will "make do" and which will need to be borrowed, rented, or

purchased—these are all decisions that visiting nurses and/or rehabilitation therapists are trained to make.

Furniture and Equipment

In setting up the sickroom, you should remove all unessential
items, so that the room will be uncluttered and easy to keep clean and
tidy. The basic furniture should include a bed, one or two bedside
tables, a chest of drawers, one straight chair, and one easy chair. All
hospital supplies should be near the patient's bed and handy. Fresh
bed linens should also be convenient. A bedtable, adjustable to
different heights, is good for eating, reading, or working on various
projects (if one is not available, a bed tray with legs works almost as
well).

If the patient enjoys television, the set should be located so that
it's easily seen from the bed. There should be a control switch that
the patient can operate himself. Having a radio and an extension
telephone at the bedside is also nice. In addition, the sickroom
should have a clock and the patient should have a bell or some
signaling device to use when he needs help. Such diversions as an
aquarium, a mobile, or interesting pictures and posters can make the
room cheerful and lively.

Of all the equipment in the sickroom, the bed is the most
important. It is difficult to give nursing care to a patient in a
full-sized double bed or one that sits low. If the patient is likely to be
in bed for a considerable period (over one month), think about
getting an electric hospital-type bed from a hospital supply store
(most communities of more than 50,000 population have one or more
hospital supply stores listed in the telephone directory under "Hospital Equipment and Supplies").

Buying an electric bed is a major expense. Depending on how
long the patient will need it, a hospital bed can also be rented or
purchased secondhand for less money. There are some voluntary
organizations that have "loan closets" of specialized as well as
sickroom equipment to be lent free of charge (call the local visiting
nurse service or the local health department to find out if your
community has such a service).

The hospital bed may be equipped with a "trapeze," which lets
the patient pull himself into a sitting position and allows certain
exercises to be done in bed. If a hospital bed is not equipped with a

trapeze, an old-fashioned "bed rope" can be used. A strong rope is fastened securely to the end of the bed and is long enough so that the patient can conveniently grasp it and pull himself to a sitting position. The hospital bed should have siderails to prevent the patient from falling out.

If the patient's illness is of short duration or you can't afford a hospital bed, you can use a twin bed as high off the floor as possible (this can be achieved by putting a platform or blocks under the bed). Make sure the elevated bed is stable. You can attach siderails to any kind of bed you use. If you need a temporary bedrail—especially for a child—you can place one side of the bed against a wall and tie the backs of tall chairs to the other side.

If you're using a regular bed and the springs are more than two years old, you should probably insert a bedboard between the springs and mattress (you can buy a commercial bedboard or use a ¾-inch slab of hard plywood cut to the appropriate size, with the edges sanded smooth). To elevate the head of a regular bed, use a number of regular pillows or place a foam-rubber wedge under the pillow.

Depending on the condition of the bedridden patient, additional bed linen will probably be needed. If the patient is thin, elderly, or has sensitive skin, special bed padding—such as sheepskin or Egg-crate padding—may be necessary to prevent bedsores.

Other Equipment

If a commode, wheelchair, or walker is needed, check the community loan closet first before renting or buying. You should also check with an occupational therapist for a recommendation on the best type of equipment for the particular patient.

It is not always necessary to purchase hospital equipment—a regular plastic bucket, for example, works better than an emesis basin, and a plastic dishpan works nicely as a bath basin. When a hospital-type urinal is not available for the male patient, use a large-mouthed plastic jar or bottle or a quart measure. If there's a handyman in the house, a commode can be made from an old straight-back chair: Cut an oval opening in the wooden seat and sand the edges of the opening carefully. Place a pail on the floor directly under the hole in the chair seat. Make a hinged cover of plywood for the seat. Take great care to keep the seat and the pail scrupulously clean to avoid odors.

There are a number of companies that specialize in home care equipment and will send a free catalog for the asking. An occupational therapist can provide you with names and addresses of such companies.

Some supplies that are used in large quantities (such as protective bed pads or gauze pads) may be ordered at wholesale prices through your doctor's office, the home health agency, or a medical supply house. Some local chapters of the American Cancer Society dispense surgical dressings and certain medications to cancer patients.

A final note: It is important that used paper tissues and other waste materials from the patient be collected and properly disposed of. This is especially important if the patient has a contagious disease, since such waste is contaminated by germs. To make a simple container, roll down the top of a lunch-sized grocery bag and pin it to the side of the bed with a large safety pin. Instruct the patient to dispose of tissues in this container. Before and after giving care to a patient, the caregiver should wash his or her hands.

Meals and Medicines

Illness often diminishes or changes appetites, so providing nourishing meals can be one of the biggest challenges for the home nurse. The following tips are meant as an introduction to this aspect of home nursing:

- Offer small portions and serve in an appealing fashion. For children, use cookie-cutters to change the shape of sandwiches. For fun salads, make faces with raw fruits and vegetables.
- Avoid salty, spicy foods but don't make the fare so bland and tasteless that it resembles hospital food.
- Unless the doctor or nurse tells you otherwise, encourage the patient to drink a variety of liquids at all hours of the day. If the patient is nauseated, offer ginger ale and ice chips. For an uncertain stomach, make liquids clear and cold and serve smaller meals more frequently.
- Use a blender to prepare soft foods or to make a variety of appetizing and nutritious concoctions. Milk shakes, fruit shakes, and soups are just a few of these.

Sometimes a patient refuses meals not because he doesn't like the food but because the consistency is unappealing. Liquid, mushy, creamy, crunchy—if possible, try to accommodate the patient's preference.

If the patient is on drug therapy at home, the caregiver should know how, when, and with what to give the medicine. For example, should medicines be given before meals? After meals? How long before or after? Should certain foods or other medicines be avoided while under medication? Should the medicine be stored in a special place? All these questions should be asked—and answered—early in the home care program.

The caregiver should establish some system to make sure that medications are given as prescribed. A medication schedule can be posted on the refrigerator door, or the amount of medicine for the day can be set out each morning and kept in a special container with times indicated.

The caregiver should keep a log of medicines taken and be prepared to show this to the doctor or nurse. If the patient refuses to take medicines because of annoying side effects, cost, religious or personal conflicts, inconvenience, or lack of understanding of what the medicine can do, this information should be shared with the nurse or physician in charge of care. Negotiating to drop certain drugs from the patient's regimen is preferable to stopping all medications without the physician's or nurse's knowledge and approval.

A Plan for Success

The physician in charge of the patient's care should provide the caregiver with explicit instructions as to the patient's condition, what type of nursing care will be required, what limitations of activity will be necessary, what the recommended diet will be, and what special treatments will be needed. *The caregiver should write these instructions down.* It's helpful to know—from the physician— how long the patient will be confined to bed and to the home (although it's often hard for anyone to make a definite prediction). Once all these facts are known, planning will be much easier.

It would be a good idea if all persons, at some time in their lives, took the 18-hour home nursing care course offered by local chapters of the American Red Cross. Knowing some of the basics of home

---

REFERENCE BOOKS THAT CAN HELP THE HOME NURSE

Brunner, Lillian Sholtis, and Doris Smith Suddarth. *Lippincott Manual of Nursing Practice*. 3d ed. New York: J. B. Lippincott Co., 1982.

Covell, Mara Brand, and Maurice Beer. *The Home Alternative to Hospitals and Nursing Homes: Creating Your Own Home Health Care Center*. New York: Rawson Associates, 1983.

Murphy, Lois Barclay. *The Home Hospital: How the Family Can Cope with Catastrophic Illness*. New York: Basic Books, 1982.

Parker, William, and Lois Dietz. *Nursing at Home*. New York: Crown Publishers, 1979.

---

nursing care can give a firm base for learning new skills as needed. Do you know, for example, how to take a patient's temperature, pulse, and respiration, or the proper way to turn a patient in bed? You should. The books listed above should prove helpful in learning some of these basic skills.

If the patient who is to receive home care needs special treatments, such as injections, dressing changes, or tracheotomy care, it would be best to call in a professional nurse for a series of teaching visits. If very complex high-tech treatments (such as respiratory therapy or intravenous therapy) are necessary, nursing and other professional services will be absolutely essential.

PROMISE OF THE FUTURE

According to one source, the growth of home health care is projected to be 40 to 50 percent per year over the next few years. The 5,000 Medicare-certified home health care agencies now in the market are only reaching 25 percent of those in need of such care. This need will increase even more as the aged population grows.

Morrie Levy, executive director of the American Federation of Home Health Agencies, sees great potential for continued expansion in the field of home health care. He explains: "The trend to earlier hospital discharge means that acutely ill patients must receive care in the home setting. Additionally, medical technology has improved to the point that many procedures—such as chemotherapy—now can be done effectively on an outpatient basis. Because of the development of new treatment techniques, which were nonexistent ten years ago, patients can receive adequate care at home and, at the same time, avoid the high cost and general dislike that characterizes hospital care."

The elderly—those over 65—are presently the greatest consumers of home health care. This is because they have more long-term diseases and other disabling health problems. Another factor is that Medicare—one of the most reliable sources of payment for certain home health services—is only available for people over 65. Private insurance companies are beginning to appreciate the advantages of home health care and are paying more generously for such services. As this trend continues, more patients under 65 will also be able to choose home care over hospital care.

Home care is significantly cheaper than institutional care, and this appeals to many third-party payers. According to the Blue Cross and Blue Shield Association, home care costs an average $50 a day, compared with the average daily hospital cost of $376.

It should be pointed out, however, that institutional care includes the cost of not only professional services and meals but also overhead and housing. Comparing costs of home versus institutional care, therefore, is like comparing apples and oranges. Furthermore, as more critically ill patients are cared for at home and require more expensive services, the cost gap between hospital and home care will narrow (although home care will probably always be cheaper).

Ten years ago the use of Foley catheters (tubes inserted in the bladder) and oxygen equipment for home care patients seemed like high technology. Now patients with tracheotomies (a tube inserted into the trachea, or windpipe, to facilitate breathing), and those receiving respiratory therapy and intravenous therapies (including antibiotic, analgesic, and hydration therapy as well as chemotherapy and nutritional feeding through a vein or a tube) can be cared for at home. In fact, almost any procedure (except major surgery) that was once limited to the hospital setting can now be carried out at home. This new technology if it's available, can shorten or prevent hospital stays for many patients.

Manufacturers and distributors of medical products and supplies have entered the field of direct service—some act as consultants to existing agencies, some have established their own home care agencies. Many different segments of the medical and business communities are finding that home care can be a healthy investment. The variety of providers that have sprung up in recent years creates competition and promotes cost effectiveness. And that can be nothing but good news for the health consumer.

Chapter 8

THINGS GO BETTER WITH FRIENDS

A real friend is someone who walks in when the rest of the world walks out.

—Walter Winchell

On an ordinary day the gift of friendship is played out in a number of ways:

- Almost every morning for the past five years, Lisa has talked with Mary on the telephone. They talk about their work, their families, their hopes, and their dreams. They also discuss their troubles and their failures.

    Mary and Lisa have seen each other at their best and their worst—there's very little one doesn't know about the other. Mary and Lisa are friends.
- For ten years Joe Lang has played softball on his company's team. When he turned 50 and his arthritis began kicking up, Joe thought he would slow the team down if he continued to play, so he told the manager he was considering quitting the team. The manager said he was speaking for the other guys: "Joe, you're a part of this team and we need you. I know Tom could use some help with the coaching—he was planning to ask you. These young guys need to work on their fielding."

    Joe Lang is fortunate to have friends who will stick with him during the good and the bad times.
- Sam and Freda Hart began having babies during the dark days of the Depression and two of their children died as

infants. One boy was born severely handicapped and lived to be only 16 years old. Their five surviving children presented Sam and Freda with many offspring and the family remained close even though two of the children moved away from the hometown.

Sam and Freda continue to live in the 50-year-old Midwestern farmhouse that they built. They putter around the place doing the chores that they're able to do. A widowed daughter lives with them.

At the time of their 60th wedding anniversary, a reporter from the local newspaper asked the Harts how they managed to stay in such good health (neither one had ever been in the hospital).

With a twinkle in her bright-blue eyes, Freda explained, "Sam and me we've seen it all and done it all."

Sam patted Freda's hand and summed it up, "There's nobody like Freda. She's my best friend."

WELL-CONNECTED
PEOPLE LEAD HEALTHIER LIVES

Friends . . . connections . . . social support systems. What's this got to do with staying health? Plenty!

Consider some results of studies published by the California Department of Mental Health (from the pamphlet "Can Friends Be Good Medicine?"):

- Women who can confide in a close friend are much less likely to become depressed.
- The rates of mental hospitalization are five to ten times greater for separated, divorced, and widowed people than for married people.
- Pregnant women under stress and without supportive relationships have three times the number of complications as pregnant women with close ties who are equally stressed.
- People who isolate themselves from others have two to three times the risk of early (premature) death.
- Terminal cancer strikes isolated people more often than it does those who are "connected."

Still not convinced? Consider a study done by Lisa F. Berkman, PhD, associate professor of epidemiology at Yale University, and

Lestor Breslow, MD, professor of public health at UCLA, who wrote the book *Health and Ways of Living*. After studying 4,725 men and women aged 30 to 60 in Alameda County, California, the researchers concluded that a person may avoid an early death if he or she is married, is a joiner of clubs, and keeps in regular contact with friends and relatives.

By caring about others, a person is more likely to take up such positive practices as exercising and to have medical checkups and health screening tests. Married people suffer less illness and have fewer accidents than those who live alone. It's for these reasons that insurance companies often increase their rates for people who become separated or divorced.

And then there's the documented connection between loneliness and heart disease. James Lynch, PhD, a leading specialist in psycho-somatic medicine from the University of Maryland School of Medicine and author of *The Broken Heart: The Medical Consequences of Loneliness*, found that the most loneliness-prone people in American society—the divorced, widowed, and elderly—are more likely to die from heart disease than other segments of the population. Loneliness, according to Dr. Lynch, is the number-one cause of premature death today.

If it's true that modern society has made us a nation of isolated individuals who subscribe to the theory of self-actualization, or "doing your own thing," maybe it's time to turn back the clock and once again discover the benefits of friends and family.

PEOPLE DO NEED PEOPLE

What Is a Friend?

A friend is one
to whom one may pour
out all the contents
of one's heart,
chaff and grain together,
knowing that the
gentlest of hands
will take and sift it,
keep what is worth keeping
and with a breath of kindness
blow the rest away.

—Arabian Proverb

A true friend is someone who cares about you and is kind to you.

For ten years, since their husbands died, Elsie Perry and Polly Nash were close church friends. They attended Sunday services, circle meetings, and women's association meetings together. They prayed for each other. When Elsie suffered a stroke and was no longer able to attend church functions, some members sent cards and some called on the phone. But it was her friend Polly who taped the minister's weekly sermons and spent every Sunday afternoon with her friend listening to the pastor's message and enjoying Sunday dinner together. Elsie and Polly always have cared about each other and have made themselves available whenever the need arose. That's another important aspect of friendship.

Tom and Joe, members of the same American Legion unit, have known each other for 20 years. Though not connected by business or family ties, they have remained loyal through the many ups and downs of their lives. They have shared many confidences and they trust each other. In addition, they have both given and received comfort from one another. These are all important qualities in a friend.

Obviously a true friend is someone very special. We all have acquaintances. But friends? They're counted on the fingers of one hand.

The dynamics of friendship have been studied for many years by great philosophers and psychologists. In the best of friendships the relationship can take on a life of its own. It's almost as though the meeting of two persons creates a new personality. The friendship becomes "us against the world," and can be one of the most powerful experiences of life. Sometimes this kind of friendship can be found in a marriage, although it's a rare individual who can have all needs met by his or her spouse. Even in a "good marriage," outside friends can enrich and bolster one's life.

Of course, no one can define what a friendship can or should mean to you. But if you find yourself lonely or if your doctor has told you that you should "get out more and meet new people," maybe it's time to begin the adventure of making a new friend.

The process of making a new friend can be described in a number of stages. First you find yourself in a place or situation where there are new people to meet. Then you share a smile, say hello, try to break down barriers. In simple terms, you get acquainted with another person. During this time, you and the acquaintance can find out if you share common experiences, interests, or activities. If you do build up a sense of commonality, friendship may progress. You may make arrangements to meet again. Depending on a number of factors, this process can move from a casual friendship to a close one or, occasionally, over a period of time, become a friendship that is deep and abiding.

THOSE STUMBLING BLOCKS

At any point in the process, the development of a friendship can be stopped or delayed.

"I never have time to meet new friends" is a common reason for avoiding involvement with others. But whatever occupies your time—work, school, family—is probably fertile ground for meeting new people. It's often not lack of time but unwillingness to make the effort to reach out to others that's the issue.

One problem that affects many older people is their physical immobility. If someone's world is limited by the walls of an apartment, there is little opportunity to make new friends. For the person who is severely handicapped or seriously ill, it's true that there may be few opportunities to "get out." Other ways must be found to keep in touch.

For many older people, however, it's not a physical infirmity that keeps them from the senior center, a club meeting, church program, or sporting event. More likely, the problem is a mild depression or the philosophy, "Why bother meeting someone else, they'll just die." This may be a time for a gentle nudge from family or friends.

One pastor has a large number of older people in his congregation. One morning he was counseling a 70-year-old member who had stopped coming to church activities. The pastor explained it this way: "A sponge will become sour if it isn't rinsed and cleansed with clean water. In the same way, a person who remains stagnant and has no interest other than self, becomes sour." This story apparently made an impression on the older parishioner, who once again joined in activities with the church.

For the person who's new in town, a good way to break the ice may be to transfer membership from a club back home to the same club in the new town. Or the person can join the local newcomer's group. Becoming active and involved is the first step in finding a friend but it does take a certain amount of energy and creativity to step outside one's usual world.

The second phase in making a friend—getting acquainted—can be painful for those who are shy. Meeting new people may make some feel like they're on display, and there's always the risk of being rejected. To compensate, some shy people develop a certain distracted or disinterested demeanor, and this can turn people away.

One bit of advice for the shy person: Try to think about the other person—who also may be shy—and think of ways to make him or her feel at ease. This will help your nervousness. When meeting someone for the first time, try to relax and reveal yourself slowly. The person who covers up shyness by being overly talkative or "coming on too strong" is as much of a turn-off as the ubiquitous wallflower.

Our friendships usually mirror our situations in life. Where we live, what we do, how we spend our leisure time sets us apart, and we generally want to make friends with those people who would feel comfortable in "our world." For these reasons, first impressions— what a person wears, how they talk—can unfortunately eliminate a considerable number of people who might be friends. Most successful friendships occur between people who are about the same age and are not in a competitive situation with one another.

Over a period of time, the testing of potential friends continues as two people get to know one another or "try each other on for fit." The more interests that friends share, the more likely the friendship will endure.

But when one considers all the possible impediments to continuing a friendship, it's a wonder that any friendships last at all. Interests change, situations change. Social mobility—either going up in the world or going down—can affect friendships. The same is true of marriage and divorce, as well as a move or the death of a friend.

To sum up, then, even though some friendships are made in heaven, most are not meant to last forever. In today's very mobile and fast-paced society, making friends is an ongoing necessity that takes time and effort.

A QUICK FIX FOR LONELINESS

Focusing on oneself and wallowing in self-pity can be detrimental emotionally and physically. Few would argue with that. But the cure may surprise you. Numerous studies point to the fact that one of the best ways to make friends and improve your emotional and physical health is to *help others*. Giving support and receiving the good feelings that come from the act is the best way to beat the blahs.

Amazing as it may seem in this sophisticated age, the old Biblical adage, "As ye sow, so shall ye reap" has never been more significant. Helping a friend or neighbor in need or volunteering in a church, hospital, school, prison, or other social service agency are all ways of "getting involved," and the process can do wonders for your morale.

Psychiatrist George Vaillant, MD, director of a 40-year study of Harvard University graduates, identified altruism as one of the qualities that helped even the most poorly adjusted men of the study group deal successfully with the stresses of life.

Wise men and women have known about altruism for years. They just may describe it differently. "It is more blessed to give than to receive" has always been a noble philosophy to guide one's life. It still is.

A LAUGH A DAY

If all this is beginning to sound too serious, I'd like to tell you a story about this traveling salesman from Omaha . . .

Jokes and laughter are good for the soul. They're also good for the body. Laughter exercises the lungs and stimulates the circulatory system. Laughter can also control pain and reduce tension.

Author Norman Cousins calls laughter a form of internal jogging and systematically used amusing books and movies to help combat his own serious ailments. Others have followed suit. Convalescent homes and hospitals bring in comedians to entertain patients and therapists use humor to treat terminally ill patients, alcoholics, drug addicts, retarded children, and depressed patients.

But no one has to get sick to discover the benefits of laughter and the importance of being around those who permit and even encourage a hearty laugh. Do you have a friend with whom you can share the silly side of life? Then nurture that friendship since it may be your lifeline to sanity and good health.

If you don't have such a friend, look around for one. But remember that a healthy sense of humor is not just laughter. Healthy humor doesn't cut down what another person *is* but what another person *does*. Healthy humor sees the light side of even serious situations. Instead of getting angry or flying off the handle, you and a friend can step back from a stressful situation and see the pretension and the humor of it. You can giggle and laugh and you'll feel better for having put some distance between you and the problem.

So stay away from negative people and find a friend that can help you lighten up your life. There may be more truth than you know in the old adage "Laugh and the world laughs with you, cry and you cry alone."

MAN'S BEST FRIEND

One deterrent to friendship—especially for men—is the old Calvinistic philosophy that a person should be self-sufficient and keep a "stiff upper lip." Obviously this type of person has difficulty making close friends.

But such a person usually allows companionship with pets, and in some cases the interaction with dogs, cats, birds, or rabbits has been extraordinarily effective in reducing loneliness and improving physical and emotional health.

A number of studies reported by Janet Davis, RN, and Anne Juhasz, PhD, in *Nursing and Health Care* substantiates the commonly held belief that pets can be therapeutic for their owners:

- In the 1800s, the Retreat at York Psychiatric Hospital in England maintained companion animals at the facility because they seemed to have a calming effect on the patients. Similarly, during World War II, the American Red Cross began pet therapy at an American Air Force convalescent center. The program proved to be beneficial, and a number of patients were allowed to take their pets with them when they were discharged from the service.
- Recent research on pet therapy has been conducted in such institutional settings as nursing homes, psychiatric hospitals, and a state prison for the criminally insane. In these studies, pets helped residents to interact and talk with others. The pets also helped to lift the patients' spirits.
- Dogs have been used successfully during therapy for emotionally disturbed children. Experience suggests that a companion animal displays unconditional acceptance and allows the child

to be in control of the situation. Communicating with a pet, therefore, is an emotionally "safe" activity for children. It can be the same for adults.

- Studies done outside institutional settings suggest that pets can have a positive effect on older people because the pets act as a bridge to other social contacts. Owning a pet gives a person something to do with his or her time and provides a ready topic of conversation.

- A correlation has been found between stroking a dog and a decrease in a person's blood pressure. Stroking an animal's fur can serve as a natural stress-reduction technique.

- The most surprising findings have been those that suggest pet ownership is an important factor in survival from cardiovascular disease. Research reported in the *Public Health Reports* showed that:

  Pet ownership, even more than marital status or family contact, emerges as an important factor in survival rates from coronary heart disease.

  For the homebound elderly person, caring for a pet can make one feel more independent. For the person who is grieving following the death of a spouse, the affection of a pet can be very comforting and healing.

  For the person who is handicapped, pets can mean the difference between staying at home and being institutionalized. There are Seeing Eye dogs for the blind and hearing dogs for the deaf. There are also dogs that can be trained to fetch and retrieve and assist people who are bedridden or wheelchair-bound.

So don't sell short the power of companion animals. It may be true, after all, that a pet can be a man's best friend.

CAN PLANTS BE MEDICINE, TOO?

Studies have shown that caring for plants can also enhance a person's physical and emotional health.

It isn't the plant itself that has any restorative powers, but it's the fact that the person who cares for the plant has a sense of responsibility for its survival. Watering the plant, fertilizing it, and monitoring its growth gives the caretaker a purpose in life. The caretaker controls the destiny of the plant, and that small act can carry over into other areas of life.

Another factor is that a plant, like an animal, can be talked to but can't talk back. That can also be therapeutic.

FRIENDS
THAT KNOW "JUST HOW YOU FEEL"

If you suddenly became a single parent, a cancer victim, or the spouse of an alcoholic, whom would you turn to for support and understanding?

Maybe you have a dear friend who could help see you through your troubled time. But would that person truly understand if he or she had never "been there"? Perhaps you would also need a friend who, by virtue of experience, could say, "I know just how you feel." Such a friend could be found most readily in a mutual-help or support group.

It's estimated that there are half a million mutual-help groups in existence. The groups fall into three categories:

1. The self-care groups for those suffering physical and mental illness (there is at least one group for nearly every major disease).
2. The reform groups for addiction behaviors (particularly the "anonymous" groups such as Alcoholics Anonymous, Gamblers Anonymous, and Overeaters Anonymous).
3. The advocacy groups for certain minorities (handicapped, elderly, mentally ill).

In all mutual-help groups there can be an overlapping of functions—self-care groups often lobby for reforms in professional care; reform groups may be involved with self-care; and minority advocacy groups may be concerned with economic and social issues.

All mutual-help groups are run *by* members *for* members and there are usually no professional salaries or overhead costs (although an office administrator or secretary is sometimes necessary).

Each group determines its own programs and schedules. Groups often hold regular meetings in church halls, public buildings, or other no-rent or low-rent facilities. Many small groups meet in members' homes. Programs for meetings might include group discussions, study groups, visiting speakers, and other activities that inform the members and help build their confidence. Some organizations publish newsletters and some maintain a hot-line service so that those in need have constant access to information and an understanding ear. Others, particularly those focusing on addictive behavior or emotional disorders, use a "buddy system," so that members can count on familiar one-on-one assistance between meetings.

There are a number of stroke clubs in the San Diego area, and the official goal of one of them is to "provide a means of resocialization and promote rehabilitation by bringing together people who have had strokes that have resulted in communication or physical difficulties."

Unofficially, each member derives different benefits from the group. Some enjoy the speakers, demonstrations, movies, and field trips; some enjoy the swapping of ideas; all enjoy the camaraderie and support that they receive from one another.

"You're with people who understand" is how Wayne Meyer feels about the stroke club. And Charlie Watkins calls the group a "morale booster—you can actually see how the other fella's getting along." For Phil Massey, joining the organization has "made me feel wanted again."

Mutual-help groups, such as a stroke club, break down the isolation that all ill or troubled people feel. They offer an atmosphere that is friendly, compassionate, and accepting. There is an unwritten code of confidentiality in such groups, and each member's privacy and dignity are respected.

All mutual-help groups have the same basic purpose: to provide emotional support and practical help in dealing with a problem common to all members. The ability to adjust to a difficult situation or life change requires *empathy* from others far more than it does *sympathy*. Mutual-help groups encourage members to share their sorrows, fears, and frustrations: From there they can begin to communicate more openly, view their problems more objectively, and find more effective coping strategies.

If you would like more information on mutual-help groups, you can look in the phone directory under the appropriate subject heading. You can also contact your local hospital, health department, or social service agency. If you're interested in a group that doesn't have a unit in your area, its central office will provide information on organizing one. Directories of mutual-help groups can be found in most public libraries, or you can write to the National Self-Help

Clearinghouse, 33 West 42nd Street, New York, NY 10036; tel. 212-840-1259.

A COMMUNITY OF FAITH

Religion is a source of strength for many people. In times of illness, they find that faith and prayer help sustain them. Many members of the clergy have completed programs that assist them in ministering to people who are ill or dying. Individual pastors can provide hope and solace, but they vary, as do doctors, nurses, and friends, in their ability to cope with life-threatening illnesses and the possibility of death.

Many pastors and church officers take on the role of instigator or coordinator of activities for patients who are physically ill or emotionally hurting. These outreach activities can include cooking, shopping, transportation, and other homemaking tasks.

Many churches are truly communities of faith that look on their parishioners as members of an extended family. When the need arises, members are ready to help each other in whatever way is necessary.

This may sound too idealistic to some, but there are many people who can attest to the goodness and helpfulness of their church family when they were ill or troubled. It's also comforting to know that when the need arises, the giver can become the receiver. The problems of one become the problems of all, and solving them becomes a community effort.

What churches have accomplished, social agencies are attempting to do. Many home care agencies and hospices, as well as hospitals, have volunteer programs. The need is great; the satisfactions are many. Service clubs—from the Boy Scouts and Girl Scouts to the Kiwanis Club—are also ready to offer assistance to members of the community. Help is frequently only a phone call away.

People need other people more than they need pills and potions, doctors and hospitals. So reach out to another person and make a friend. It could be the most important thing you ever do.

Chapter 9

HEALTH MAINTENANCE ORGANIZATIONS— THE WAVE OF THE FUTURE

Forty-one-year-old Paul Masters was an avid tennis player who kept in shape during the week by playing basketball at the YMCA near his office. It was during one lunch-hour game that he slipped, turned his ankle, and felt a terrible surge of pain up his right leg. A friend drove him to the emergency room, where x-rays were taken and he was seen by an orthopedist, Dr. Craig. The diagnosis: a broken bone in the ankle. A plaster cast was applied and Paul was taught how to walk with crutches.

It was spring, and Paul hoped for a quick recovery so that he could be back on the tennis courts by summer. But it didn't work out that way.

Every month Paul saw Dr. Craig and had an x-ray taken. After three months the bones had not pulled together and Dr. Craig discussed the possibility of surgical pinning. Paul, an engineer, wondered about the use of electromagnetic therapy (electromagnetic fields accelerate bone growth). Dr. Craig didn't discount either possibility but wanted to continue the cast for a while longer. He prescribed extra vitamin D and calcium to aid healing.

Another month went by and summer arrived. The one-piece plaster cast was hot, so it was replaced with a bivalve (two-piece) fiberglass cast. This could be removed, and Paul was able to soak his leg regularly. Finally, toward the end of the summer the x-ray showed that there was a union of the bones, and a bivalve walking cast was applied. The crutches were put aside and Paul was able to play a little golf. Six weeks later, when the walking cast was also put aside, Paul started activities slowly. Six months later he was back on the tennis courts, grateful that surgery had not been necessary and satisfied with the treatment he received during his long illness.

Unfortunately, surgery can't always be avoided. Nine-year-old Sarah Haig had suffered for years from middle-ear infections. Unlike her brothers and sisters, though, there seemed to be no warning for her. One minute her right ear would feel "funny," and the next minute a mixture of blood and pus would ooze out of it. These were sure signs of a serious middle-ear infection and a ruptured eardrum. Sarah's pediatrician was concerned. Antibiotics healed the infection—temporarily—but there was a permanent hole in her eardrum, and this would have to be repaired by microscopic surgery. Sarah was referred to an ear, nose, and throat (ENT) doctor.

At first it seemed like a wonderful adventure—the idea of going to the hospital, having surgery, and getting all that attention. But Sarah and her parents were scared too, and the ENT doctor (who would perform the operation) discussed all the details of surgery with them.

Sarah and her mother went to an afternoon program that the hospital sponsored for kids who were going to the hospital. They were shown a movie about hospitalization and then they got to try on and play with such equipment as the anesthesia mask, the surgical "hat," blood pressure cuff, and emesis basin. The children were encouraged to ask questions and express their feelings.

Sarah was admitted to the hospital on the day of surgery. During the operation, she was not allowed to see family members, but on the night of surgery Sarah's mother sat in a chair by her bed. Sarah had a bad night, and her mother was glad to be there to help her. The next day Sarah went home to recuperate. A week later she was back in school. Gradually, Sarah's hearing returned to normal and the ear problem was quickly forgotten.

A year later, however, during a routine checkup with her pediatrician, it was apparent that the graft had given way and that the surgery would have to be repeated. It was not a happy time for Sarah, her family, or the surgeon, but all knew what to expect, and

Sarah's mother again spent that first night after surgery in a lounge chair beside Sarah's hospital bed. The surgery and recuperative period went smoothly.

Two years later the new eardrum is intact, and Sarah can hear well. She continues to see the ENT doctor twice a year. Except for the fact that she can't dive, Sarah is able to do everything else that children her age do. Because both of her hospital stays were short(overnight) and her mother was able to stay with her, Sarah does not remember her hospitalization as a "bad experience." Her parents couldn't have been happier with the type of care they chose for their daughter.

Shortly after she moved with her family from the East to the West Coast, 38-year-old Eileen Wilson found herself pregnant for the seventh time. Two of her pregnancies had ended in miscarriages, but she had four healthy children at home.

When she was six weeks pregnant, Eileen went for her first visit with the obstetrician. At this time, Eileen brought up *her* concerns about her age and the safety of having another baby. The possibility of amniocentesis was discussed and strongly advised by the obstetrician. (Amniocentesis is a procedure whereby a sample of amniotic fluid, which surrounds the baby during intrauterine life, is obtained by puncturing the amniotic sac through the abdomen. It is used in the prenatal diagnosis of certain disorders, such as Down's syndrome and many hereditary metabolic diseases.)

Eileen agreed to think about having the procedure done, but really wasn't too keen on it for several reasons. First, since she had already suffered two miscarriages, she felt that she was at some increased risk to miscarry again just by having the procedure. More important, if the amniocentesis did show that the baby was defective in some way, she wasn't prepared to have an abortion. It was morally repugnant to her. Before her next obstetrical visit, a genetic counselor called and discussed the whole issue with Eileen. With an appreciation of the risks involved, the 38-year-old mother decided not to have amniocentesis. "I decided to put my faith in God rather than the medical establishment to assure that all would turn out well."

But Eileen wasn't foolish. She followed a sensible diet, exercised regularly, and got adequate rest. She never missed an obstetrical appointment and looked forward especially to visits with the nurse practitioners who offered her practical sugggestions and emotional support. Eileen decided not to attend Lamaze classes, although these were offered to her. The time was not convenient, and besides, "I've been through all that before."

When the time came for the baby to be born, the labor did not move along as quickly as might have been expected. The baby was large, and after 12 hours of active labor, medication was given to speed things along. The doctors and nurses were concerned and attentive. Soon a ten-pound girl was delivered. She was normal and healthy in every way. Eileen and her family were grateful for the fine care that had been given. Eileen was especially glad that the kind of care she selected allowed her to do some things *her* way.

Eileen, Paul, and Sarah could have received similar medical care in almost any major city in the country. But the truth is that all three live in San Diego and are members of Kaiser Permanente, the nation's largest health maintenance organization.

Following Eileen's pregnancy and delivery, and after Sarah's two surgeries, the only bill they received was a small charge for use of the hospital telephone. Paul had to pay for the crutches he used, but all other expenses were paid for by Kaiser, and there were no medical reimbursement forms to fill out.

When the Wilson, Masters, and Haig families signed on with Kaiser, they knew their entire family could use the Kaiser facilities whenever it was necessary. If they needed treatment that couldn't be provided by a Kaiser facility, the health plan would send them to another hospital and Kaiser would pay the bill. If any of the family members became ill or were injured in another city, the plan would pay for emergency care.

All this may sound too good to be true. But in today's over-priced, fragmented medical care system, health maintenance organizations may be an idea whose time has come.

Health maintenance organizations, or HMOs, combine prepayment with a group practice that provides comprehensive medical care. What this means to the health consumer is that all health and medical care—except dental care—is provided by one organization that charges a flat monthly premium rather than charging for each service, each office visit, each surgery. Members don't have to choose doctors and hospitals, file claims, or wait to be reimbursed.

HMOs have grown spectacularly in recent years—from 72 enrolling 4.4 million people in 1973, when the federal government began pushing HMO membership, to about 300 covering 14 million people today.

In spite of opposition by many physicians, HMOs seem to be making a foothold. What events led up to today's popularity?

HOW IT ALL BEGAN

At the turn of the century, medical care in this country was primarily given by general practitioners in solo practices. Fees were paid for services rendered. Some years later, third-party payments by insurance companies helped to assure that doctors would be paid. However, a survey by *Medical Economics* in 1933 showed that private practitioners were collecting only about 40 percent of the fees they charged. Physicians seemed to take this as a matter of course. They were allowed to practice as they saw fit, with little interference from government agencies or outside forces. Medical care in those days, of course, was less complex than it is today. But even before the days of specialization and high technology, there were some who had revolutionary ideas about how the medical industry could be run.

In the late 1920s and early 1930s—the time of the Depression— some significant changes occurred. Specifically, three group-practice prepayment plans were formed that became the predecessors of today's HMOs.

In 1929 Michael Shadid, MD, established the Farmer's Union Co-operative Hospital Association in Elk City, Oklahoma. Its goal was to help farmers obtain comprehensive, quality medical care in a cost-effective manner through a cooperative arrangement.

About the time of Shadid's experiment, employees of the Los Angeles Department of Water and Power arranged for two physicians, Donald Ross and Clifford Loos, to provide comprehensive hospital and medical services for about 2,000 workers and their dependents. By 1935 the Ross-Loos Clinic had enrolled more than 37,000 members. (In 1980 Ross-Loos was purchased by a large insurance firm, but it continues to grow with no change in its basic mode of operation.)

Also in 1929, in the Mojave Desert, Sidney Garfield, MD, and his colleagues were providing medical care on a prepaid basis to 5,000 workers building an aqueduct that would carry water to Los Angeles. This service caught the attention of one of the contractors, Henry J. Kaiser, and in 1937 he persuaded Dr. Garfield to provide a similar service to the work force at the Grand Coulee Dam. This was the beginning of the Kaiser Permanente Medical Care Program, which today serves 4.4 million members.

Later, in 1937, federal employees of the Home Owners' Loan Corporation in Washington, D.C., formed the Group Health Association of America (GHAA), a group-practice prepayment plan that exists today and serves 110,000 members in the Washington, D.C., area. Organized medicine actively opposed this first urban plan by making it difficult for GHAA physicians to join the local medical association and obtain staff privileges in local hospitals. This conflict led to battles in the courts and slow but steady victories for HMOs.

The basic concepts for prepaid group practice that guided these early efforts and that sustain the HMO industry today consist of six basic principles, or "The Genetic Code." They are:

- Group practice.
- Integration of facilities, meaning combining both outpatient and hospital facilities, to get maximum utilization of equipment and personnel.
- Prepayment.
- Preventive medicine, which emphasizes keeping the patient well as much as treating the sick.
- Voluntary enrollment, which enables those who don't like the prepaid group practice format to choose an alternative type of plan.
- Physician responsibility for patient care as well as planning, financing and allocation of resources.

In 1970 Paul Ellwood, MD, who coined the term health maintenance organization, helped develop the policy statement that led to federal legislation for the establishment of HMOs. In 1973 Congress passed the Health Maintenance Organization Act. Besides providing federal grants and loans for new HMOs, it set aside restrictive state laws, granting federal qualification to any HMO that met specific requirements. The 1973 law also required that every company with more than 25 employees had to offer the HMO option if an HMO offered its services.

The entrance of such insurance giants as Prudential and INA (Insurance Company of North America) into the HMO field further proves that HMOs are considered worthy investments for some entrepreneurs.

And, aided by government support, the number of HMOs has steadily been growing in major cities across the country. However, in

1982 it was estimated that about half the U.S. population lived in cities or rural areas without an HMO.

LOW COST, LESS HOSPITALIZATION

Critics (particularly physicians) have frequently charged that HMOs save money by enrolling younger, healthier people who don't need much care. The recent federally financed Rand Corporation study shows that this accusation is untrue. It suggests instead that HMOs save money *by avoiding hospitalization,* the most expensive kind of care. The Rand study, one of the best of its kind, was conducted as follows:

A total of 1,580 volunteers—individuals as well as families—were randomly assigned to get free care for three to five years in one of two ways: either traditional fee-for-service care from any physicians they chose or membership in a large HMO, the Group Health Cooperative of Puget Sound.

Also studied were another 733 Group Health members who were already enrolled and 782 persons paying for part of the fee-for-service care, just as they would pay for health insurance. The two groups—HMO patients and traditional doctors' patients—were equally matched for health, age, sex, race, family size, and income.

Results showed that the HMO members had 40 percent fewer hospital admissions and days in the hospital than the fee-for-service patients, and their total care cost 28 percent less. The HMO doctors practiced a less costly style of medicine than fee-for-service (largely solo practice) physicians.

"In an HMO," says Willard Manning, head of the Rand team, "the economic incentive is strong to keep patients out of hospitals. This is because the HMO acts as both health care provider and insurer. . . . When hospital costs go up, premiums have to be raised . . . and the HMO begins to lose members."

Previous studies have demonstrated that HMOs offer more extensive ambulatory care, thus increasing demand for these services. In addition, if there is a choice between providing care on either an inpatient or outpatient basis, the HMO will probably choose the less costly outpatient mode. All this adds up to less hospitalization and a more cost-effective way of providing medical care.

Another point to be considered: As mentioned in chapter 1, there are many important reasons why a person should avoid going to the hospital to begin with. In an HMO, where total care is promised, the organization has to live with any mistakes it makes. If it is a fact that performing a hysterectomy on a woman is going to result in a number of postsurgical problems (and the HMO will have to care for these problems), it makes sense for the HMO physicians to pursue every other avenue before taking up the scalpel.

Does this mean, then, that HMO physicians undertreat their patients—sending them on a round of second, third, and fourth opinions before finally coming to some decision? No. The best bet is that the conservative approach of HMOs is a good one for the patient, whereas the overtreatment by some fee-for-service physicians is not in the best interest of the patient. Further studies are now under way that will determine exactly how HMOs reduce hospital admissions by 40 percent.

The Rand project, conducted from 1976 to 1981, and reported in 1984, is particularly significant since the HMO members who were studied had become members by choice. Many were state and federal employees and University of Washington faculty members. The style and quality of the HMO obviously appealed to this well-educated, middle-income group.

OTHER HEALTH CARE CHOICES

So, if HMOs are perceived to be the salvation of the medical industry and most customers are satisfied with the care they receive, why haven't they grown more rapidly? One definite reason is the antagonism of the medical profession that started in the 1940s and persists to this day. Fee-for-service physicians are threatened economically by HMOs and have fought back by attacking the type of medical care that HMOs provide.

In some areas of the country, however, physicians have elected not to "fight 'em" but to "join 'em." Fee-for-service physicians, faced with the loss of a substantial number of patients, have themselves formed a type of HMO called the independent practice association, or IPA. IPAs are rising fast because they are more acceptable to many doctors and patients, although they may not be as efficient as HMOs.

In a typical IPA, a large group of physicians band together, contract with hospitals to provide medical services at a fixed daily rate, then offer a prepaid group plan to employee groups similar to those who join more traditional HMOs. Doctors belonging to IPAs usually treat both fee-for-service patients and prepaid group patients.

In Minnesota there's an IPA called Physicians Health Plan. The November/December 1982 issue of *American Health* reported on this group, which offered the choice of more than 200 physicians in a 13-county area. The IPA physicians treated patients in their own offices for one fixed premium that was usually all-inclusive and paid for by patients or their employers.

Physicians in the IPA had a collective stake in keeping costs down. They received only 80 percent of their usual fees until the plan broke even. So they imposed tough rules on themselves. They let IPA executives withhold payment from any physician who sent a non-emergency patient to the hospital without a "preadmission certification" of need from an IPA nurse, who also approved the planned duration of stay. If the patient stayed longer than the nurse allowed, someone from the IPA called the hospital daily to check on that patient's progress.

IPAs may offer more personalized service than a typical HMO, but IPAs often have no centralized facility and may not have a firm administration that insists on cost-cutting efficiencies. An IPA, therefore, probably won't offer as many advantages as an HMO.

The competition of HMOs has encouraged some doctors outside the system to develop still another way to provide health care. Some fee-for-service doctors, outpatient clinics, and even hospitals have formed preferred provider organizations (PPOs). These charge less than the competition for medical treatment or rely less on such costly treatments as surgery. Incentives may take the form of reduced or eliminated deductibles for policy hospitals that use preferred providers.

One example of a PPO is the California Blue Cross System called the Prudent Buyer Plan. Blue Cross, with four million state subscribers, has already contracted with 9,000 of California's 55,000 doctors and 136 of its 530 hospitals to provide service at lower "preferred" cost. Eventually Blue Cross expects to sign up a third of the state's doctors. Blue Cross patients who see one of the other two-thirds will still be covered. But they'll have to pay the cost difference out of their own pockets.

PPOs are outlawed in some states and are unregulated. There is also some confusion over their definition.

HMOs, IPAs, PPOs—today's health consumer can drown in a sea of alphabet soup. Some patients—particularly Medicare patients—have signed up with these new programs only to find that the quality is not what they had expected, or that the company very quickly went bankrupt and they were left with substantial medical bills.

One Florida-based HMO, International Medical Center (IMC), served 120,000 patients in the Miami and Tampa areas. Ninety thousand of these patients were senior citizens who "turned in" their Medicare cards and agreed to let the HMO provide their total medical care. The government was watching closely to see if this would be a feasible way to reduce sky-rocketing costs for Medicare patients (the HMO had agreed to charge Medicare 5 percent less than the usual patient cost). In 1984 IMC suffered financial problems and planned to merge with Miami General Hospital. State insurance officials feared that the company was covering up serious financial problems and ordered it to hand over records so that its financial soundness could be evaluated. However, according to newspaper accounts, IMC was cleared and is still in business.

As more HMOs spring up around the country, they will be subjected to this same scrutiny by both public officials and consumers. Time will tell which ones will survive in the increasingly competitive health care business.

THE PROS OF HMOs

From a personal point of view, there are both advantages and disadvantages to joining an HMO. Using Kaiser (where my family and I have been members since 1977) as a model, some of the advantages are immediately apparent:

Coordinated Care—Medical services and records are in one place. Physicians, ancillary personnel, laboratories, diagnostic facilities, and pharmacy are often located in one central spot, with satellite clinics in additional locations. One-stop health care service is not only convenient, but it makes good sense medically, since all your care can be coordinated. Diagnostic tests need not be duplicated, and there is less chance of drug reactions going undetected because all health workers know what care is being provided. A number of physicians will have access to your health records and can provide a system of "checks and balances" on the health care you receive.

Economic Security—All medical and surgical care, hospitalization, diagnostic and laboratory tests, and x-rays are paid for in advance when you join most HMOs. Some allow a reduction on pharmacy costs. However, there are some variations that need to be pointed out. If a patient joins Kaiser, for example, as an individual rather than through his employer, there will be a slight fee each time he or she sees a doctor. Some private insurance companies that offer HMOs require patients to pay a deductible fee and also a percentage of certain costs. Generally speaking, though, even with the deductible and co-payment provisions, HMOs are cheaper than the traditional fee-for-service system.

Additional Services—Because of the emphasis that Kaiser and some other HMOs place on preventive medicine, there are many programs that are offered free of charge to its members. These will be discussed in greater detail later in this chapter.

Quality Care—Fee-for-service physicians have frequently charged that HMOs give less than quality care to their patients. But this has not been supported by the several major studies that have been done on HMOs. In 1980 John Williamson, MD, and Francis Cunningham of Johns Hopkins School of Hygiene and Public Health reviewed 27 studies comparing care received by HMO members with care received by a similar group in the fee-for-service system. They concluded that, "in 19 studies, the investigators found the quality of care in HMOs to be superior to that in other settings." In the other eight studies, quality of care was found to be similar or the findings were not conclusive. In none of the studies was the quality of HMO care found to be below that of fee-for-service care.

Another 1980 study was conducted by the American Medical Association's Council on Medical Service. The AMA looked at earlier HMO studies and also conducted its own review of 15 HMOs representing a cross section of size, location, and date of onset. The council concluded: "To the extent that various factors used in quality assessment have been used to measure care for HMO enrollees and for a comparable fee-for-service population, the medical care delivered by the HMOs appears to be of a generally high quality. . . . The

HMO approach, where viable, appears to have the potential to provide health care of acceptable quality at a lower total cost to enrollees than many other health care systems." The AMA group also found that "nothing in the literature indicates that HMO savings result from enrollees receiving less care than they need."

HMOs, however, are not for everyone. There are some definite drawbacks that must be considered.

If it's important to you to be able to walk or drive a short distance to receive medical care, an HMO might not be your best bet. To be cost effective, large HMOs have centralized facilities and this may mean extra travel and some inconvenience. In terms of overall efficiency and cost savings, however, the extra traveling is usually worth it.

A more important consideration is that if you already have a satisfactory relationship with a fee-for-service physician, it would not be in your best interest to join an HMO, because that personal relationship would have to be severed or you would have to pay out of pocket to continue being seen by that special physician.

It is possible, in both a large and a small HMO, to have your own physician. Regular visits and most "sick" visits can be arranged with a physician of your choice, and a relationship of trust can be developed just as it is with a private practice physician. And if you don't like a particular physician, you are usually free to choose another.

However, the HMO physician you choose will probably not be available in an emergency unless he's "on call," and you may not be able to get through to "your doctor" on the telephone. For some patients that may be a real problem.

If you are truly ill, my experience has been that quality of care is never compromised at an HMO. But often the personal touch, the relaxed bedside manner, may be missing. As one patient put it, "An HMO is run by triage—the sick are always cared for promptly and adequately. But the walking well won't be pampered. If you like having someone always hold your hand, you probably won't be satisfied in an HMO."

The elitist patient might feel that an HMO smacks of working-class or welfare clinics, although in actual practice this is far from the truth—but the stigma may seem real to some.

"I don't want everybody knowing my business" is another frequent complaint and certainly a valid one, since your health records may go through the hands of many physicians and health workers. If privacy is a real issue for you, that may be another reason for saying no to a large, impersonal HMO.

Another drawback is the long waiting time for non-urgent appointments (up to two months for a routine eye examination or one month to see a dermatologist for acne treatment). In addition, some specialists can be consulted only after the patient is seen by the primary care provider (internist, family physician, pediatrician, nurse practitioner, or physician assistant). Suppose, for example, a young athlete has a chronic knee problem that she feels should be seen by an orthopedist. The young woman could not make an appointment directly with an orthopedist, but would have to be seen first by her primary care physician, who would refer her, if necessary, to the orthopedist. The same is true when consulting an ear, nose, and throat physician or a surgeon. In an emergency, of course, the patient is immediately seen by the appropriate specialist.

ONE DOCTOR WHO CARED

Some feel that HMOs provide impersonal care. But many fee-for-service physicians are cold and indifferent and keep patients waiting far too long. Most HMOs are now making a real effort to give more individualized and personal care to their clients. One story, which appeared in a May 1984 issue of the *San Diego Union,* bears repeating (the names have been charged).

Emily Bridgeman carried a tiny infant in her arms when she kept her appointment with the physician on call at the Kaiser facility in Southern California. Emily, mother of three young children, was in her early 30s and had recently been suffering from severe chest pains. The Kaiser physician ("Dr. Jim") who saw Emily reviewed her chart and found that two years before she had had a melanoma—a malignant mole—removed from her leg. When Dr. Jim saw Emily's chest x-ray from this visit, it showed that the melanoma had spread to the lungs. Emily and her family were, of course, shocked and saddened by the news. The young Dr. Jim was too. In fact, Emily's case changed the way he now practices medicine.

When Emily came to the urgent appointment clinic, Dr. Jim was moved by the young woman's spirit and the enormousness of her problem. Since the young physician lived nearby and had vacation time coming, he decided to visit Emily's home from time to time. He checked on her medical progress and offered spiritual encouragement and prayed with her. In three months Emily Bridgeman died. At the time of her death, Emily's husband and Dr. Jim were at her bedside. The entire experience made a lasting impression on the young Kaiser physician. He now works more closely with all his patients and becomes involved with them—a concept that many find atypical in the vast maze of the Kaiser Permanente health facilities.

Not every HMO has a Dr. Jim on staff, but many prepaid health plans know they must give more personalized and humanistic care if they are to survive in the very competitive health care industry. Because Kaiser offers so many advantages to physicians, there is often a waiting list of those who want to be on staff. HMOs are frequently in the position to pick the "best and brightest."

Generally speaking, HMOs do best in growing areas (the Sun Belt, for example), where new residents don't have established ties with a physician and are willing to accept a different concept in medical care.

HOW COMMUNITIES
CAN ORGANIZE CARE

If you think an HMO might be something you'd like to join, your first step is to see if one exists in your community. If you work, you can talk to the benefits administrator or a union representative at your place of employment. Companies who have 25 or more employees and offer health insurance as a benefit are required to give their employees the option of joining a federally qualified HMO if there is one in the community. In investigating an HMO program, you might ask the company representative if HMO members are generally satisfied and if their numbers are growing. You may want to talk with some members.

If you're retired or working in a small business, you may also join an HMO as an individual (if there are openings). For a list of HMOs in your state, you can write to the Information Department, Group Health Association of America, 624 Ninth Street, NW, Washington, DC 20001.

Assuming that there is an HMO near your home, you should consider the following guidelines before joining:

Federally Qualified?—Federal qualification requires that an HMO offer a wide range of care, including short-term mental health services, treatment for alcoholism and drug abuse, home health care, family planning, and health education programs. Federal qualification also means that the HMO agrees to various regulations that protect its members (such as formal grievance procedures to get problems resolved quickly and effectively). All this is good news from the health consumer's point of view. However, some excellent HMOs, for one reason or another, have chosen not to become federally qualified.

Member, Group Health Association of America (GHAA)—Membership in this group gives some indication of financial soundness. By writing to this organization (address on page 146), you can find out which HMOs are federally qualified and which are members of GHAA. The association has certain standards that members must abide by and takes pride in the fact that, even if one of their members becomes insolvent, no individual has ever been left without medical coverage or been responsible for medical bills.

Facilities—What services does the HMO in your community provide? Are the offices, hospital, and emergency services convenient to your home? Are the laboratory, diagnostic, and pharmacy departments in a centralized location or inconveniently scattered about? Are there facilities for educational and preventive medicine programs?

If you're considering joining an IPA (independent practice association, run by physicians at a cost savings to patients), you may receive more individualized service than you would in a typical HMO, but an IPA may not offer the advantages of a consolidated facility and closely managed organization. With an IPA, you may end up in a situation that is more expensive and fragmented than in a typical HMO.

Reputation—How old is the HMO you're considering and what is its track record? Who backs the HMO—a large insurance company, a union, a hospital, or a group of physicians? If possible, check the financial solvency of the HMO owner.

Generally speaking, an older established HMO is a better bet than a new one. Because of poor management and skimpy capitalization, some new HMOs don't survive and leave members high and dry.

Finally, talk to other members. Are they satisfied with the HMO they've chosen? Do they find the service impersonal or are there long waits?

Credentials of HMO Physicians—Does the roster of HMO physicians read like a membership list in the United Nations? If there is a *majority* of foreign physicians on staff, this *may* indicate inferior schooling and communication problems with patients.

Some HMOs will give prospective members a list of their medical staff with background information. It's always a good recommendation if the HMO's physicians are board certified in their specialties (which means they've passed certain tests in that specialty) or at least board eligible (which means they've completed the required residency but have not yet passed the test for their specialty). One study by the AMA found that most physicians in HMOs *were* board certified.

Some Other Considerations—Is there a high turnover of physicians or have most been on staff for a number of years? Is there a mix of older and younger physicians?

SETTING TRENDS FOR THE FUTURE

Regardless of whether you have the option of becoming an HMO member or even choose to join one, there is much to be learned from the organization's innovative concepts. Many features of HMOs are being borrowed by more traditional health care providers. As an informed health consumer, you should be aware of some of the trends that HMOs began:

Lowered Hospital Admissions—As mentioned earlier, HMOs attain their greatest amount of savings by keeping their patients *out* of the hospital. Using Kaiser as an example, the cost and utilization chart for 1981 on page 149 (reprinted with permission from the California Health Facilities Commission) shows how much savings is involved.

Within the non-HMO population, public program beneficiaries account for a disproportionately high utilization of inpatient care. After removing these high utilizers from both populations, the study found HMO hospital use to be lower, at 328 patient days per 1,000 versus 565 in non-HMO hospitals (these are the "adjusted" data).

What accounts for the lowered hospitalization rate in HMOs? It isn't because HMO members are any healthier. The reason is that many surgical procedures and tests are performed on an outpatient,

	HMO	Non-HMO
Cost		
Cost per person per year	$ 177	$ 459
Cost per hospital day	$ 429	$ 453
Cost per hospital stay	$2,381	$3,068
Utilization		
Admissions per 1,000 per year	74	149
Patient days per 1,000 per year	413	1,012
Average length of stay in days	5.6	6.8

or ambulatory, basis. Hospitalization is the last resort.

Traditional medical insurance plans normally cover more of a patient's medical bill if the patient is in the hospital than if the patient receives the same care in the doctor's office. For this reason, fee-for-service doctors are more likely to hospitalize their patients. An HMO, on the other hand, knows that it costs more for hospitalization (a bill that it must pay), so if the patient can safely be treated outside the hospital, that's the way it will be done.

Another consideration: Surgeons who are on the staff of an HMO receive the same salary regardless of whether they do four surgeries a day or ten. Unless it's medically necessary, they have no economic incentive to do unnecessary surgery (just as the internist has no economic incentive to put the patient in the hospital for tests).

Greater Use and Popularity of Nurse Practitioners and Physician Assistants as Primary Health Care Providers—Not every patient who walks into a doctor's office really needs the skills of a highly trained physician. Many patients need someone to evaluate their medical problem, but more important, they need someone to listen to them, talk to them, and help educate and reassure them. This job is often done best by a nurse practitioner (NP) or physician assistant (PA) at considerable savings to the patient (the average physician's salary at an HMO is $60,000, while the average salary of a nurse practitioner or physician assistant is $22,000).

HMOs have found these health workers to be highly successful and popular with patients. Exactly how many do they employ?

Recent statistics from Kaiser indicate that for every 100,000 members, approximately 100 physicians are employed. Keeping these figures constant, the number of nurse practitioners and physician assistants who work as primary care providers varies from area to area:

Area	No. of PAs and NPs per 100,000 Members
Connecticut	42.0
Colorado	33.3
Oregon	20.5
Washington, D.C.	17.3
Texas	17.0
Southern California	16.2
Ohio	14.7
Hawaii	10.7
Northern California	7.2

The use of nurse practitioners and physician assistants varies from region to region because of state laws that apply. In addition, in areas where Kaiser facilities are just starting up, there tends to be a higher ratio of nurse practitioners and physician assistants. Once the facility is established, the ratio goes down.

Kaiser also has a Nurse Anesthetist School in Los Angeles, and the use of the nurse anesthetists—supervised by an MD anesthesiologist—is increasing.

Who are these "super nurses" and "assistant doctors" and what can they do?

A nurse practitioner is an RN who has received additional education—ranging from six months to two years—at a school of nursing or medical college, or at a hospital or agency in conjunction with a college or university. Both the National League for Nursing and the American Nurses' Association encourage graduate education (master's degree in nursing) for the preparation of nurse practitioners, although at the present time there is no standardization of programs or national examination to demonstrate competency. Nurse practitioner programs provide additional knowledge and skills in areas that were once considered to be solely in the physician's domain. They can, and often do, handle about 80 percent of the cases.

What exactly can a nurse practitioner do? She is able to take a medical history, do a physical examination, order diagnostic tests, and treat the patient's immediate problem. She can also assess the patient's emotional status and direct an overall health plan that would include prevention of disease and disability.

Do patients get second-class care when they're seen by nurses rather than doctors? Quite the contrary. A study conducted at the University of Manitoba, Canada, showed that nurses can be *more* successful than doctors in treating certain patients. The university had two clinics for hypertensive (high blood pressure) patients—one was run by nurses and the other by physicians. The nurses were more successful in controlling obesity, a major factor in hypertension. The study revealed that nurses scheduled more appointments than the MDs did, and the nurses followed up on their patients more closely when supervising therapy.

The doctors, on the other hand, referred nearly half their patients to hospital dieticians. Even though the nurses did not have the skilled training of the dieticians, the nurses were more successful with their patients.

Nurses (and nurse practitioners) provide a particularly personal kind of care. They often pick up on psychological cues or social problems that can delay a patient's progress. Patients frequently ask nurses "stupid" questions—questions that they would never ask their doctors.

Nursing and medical philosophies are quite different. Nurses focus on keeping patients well, or if they are sick, comforting and educating them about health. Physicians, on the other hand, generally concentrate on illness.

Nurse practitioners know their limits, however. They don't perform surgery or do involved diagnostic evaluations. They work under established medical protocol and always have a physician nearby who can provide additional expertise for more serious medical problems.

Physician assistants are also used as primary health care providers in HMOs. But, though they may perform tasks similar to those done by nurse practitioners, physician assistants are very different.

The training for a PA is usually two years in a medical school-based program, and the curriculum is concentrated on medical subjects. According to the Association of Physician Assistant Programs, almost 90 percent of PA students have had health care experience before entering the program, and almost one-half hold associate degrees or bachelor of science degrees.

The "typical" PA is an older person with some medical background and/or training (in the beginning, many medics and corpsmen from the armed services became physician assistants). Initially, more men than women entered PA programs. At the present time, 60 percent of physician assistants are men and 40 percent are women, but the students entering educational programs are now balanced 50-50.

Physician assistants perform such functions as taking histories, doing physical examinations, and often diagnosing and treating patients—all under the direction of a physician.

To many physicians (even in an HMO), physician assistants are more palatable than nurse practitioners. This is because PAs are in a more closely defined and controlled role. Nurse practitioners are more autonomous and do tasks outside the scope of medicine. This can be threatening to physicians.

Importance of Preventive Care—Health education has been provided by Kaiser for many years. Traditionally the program has sought to provide patients who suffer from a variety of chronic conditions with opportunities to learn about their illness, so they could participate more fully and knowledgeably in their own care. Some newer programs represent an effort to move beyond patient education to interventions that will prevent disease and promote good health.

In Kaiser's Southern California region, for example, 4,000 members have been treated in the antismoking program. Sixty percent of those who complete the program don't smoke two years after treatment (according to Kaiser officials, this is roughly twice the success rate of other efforts, as reported in the professional literature). The program, which uses a combination of behavior modification techniques, consists of five consecutive treatment sessions and 14 maintenance sessions over a 12-month period. The program is presently available to all Kaiser members in the Southern California region, with no additional charge, and is being established in other Kaiser medical centers.

In Ohio there is a program to help overweight children. In San Diego there is one for overweight adults. In Oregon and at the Fontana Medical Center in the Southern California region, alcohol abuse programs were conducted which tested the proposition that detoxification could be handled effectively outside the hospital. In San Jose, California, Kaiser, in cooperation with two local colleges, offers its members a number of courses designed for "More Effective Living." The topics range from obesity, insomnia, and "How to Handle Stress" to "Managing Money for Health."

Obviously, Kaiser is not the only HMO in this country and, in fact, its facilities only touch a small portion of the total population receiving health care. Because of space limitations, it is impossible to describe all health maintenance plans. Kaiser is highlighted because it is an example of a well-established, well-operated HMO. It's also the largest in the country and is often used as a model for health maintenance organizations that are just forming.

Chapter 10
CARE &
THE MENTALLY ILL

Care of the mentally ill in this country is a social scandal. Consider the following:

- In April 1985, a Senate investigation revealed that mentally ill patients in state-run institutions are subject to such abuses as neglect, intimidation, sexual advances, and rape, as well as kicking and striking by personnel.

  The six-month subcommittee investigation looked at 31 institutions in 12 states. It was found that these facilities provided little treatment other than prescribed medication, and many failed to maintain even decent living conditions.

  One 12-year-old boy, for example, was injured 124 times while a patient in a state institution, although his parents were informed of only 25 such "incidents." As a result of his injuries, the boy has lost the use of his right arm and leg and has generally lost many skills he possessed before being confined to the institution.

  A mentally retarded patient in another state institution was caged in a shower room seven days a week, 24 hours a day, and let out only at mealtimes. Fortunately the young man was released to a group home and is now doing well.

- A 30-year-old Southern California man died of a drug over-dose after he was admitted to a community mental health facility. According to reports, the man was not given a thorough examination but was placed in restraints and seclusion, where he subsequently died.
- Across America men and women spend nights huddled in apartment hallways and deserted buildings or skulking around in filthy alleyways. Many spend their days in public libraries or train stations. They bathe their lice-infested bodies and wash their clothes in the public bathroom sinks and drag their bedrolls and duffel bags wherever they go. Many frequent the "soup kitchens," and some sell empty bottles and cans to buy a little food or cheap liquor.

    These are the "street people" of America, and about half of them are mentally ill. Some are potentially violent—most are fragile and out of touch. A significant number end up in jail charged with everything from nuisance offenses to very violent acts against society. All need a safe place to live, but in most communities no such place exists.

These are no longer the days of *One Flew Over the Cuckoo's Nest,* where frontal lobotomies were a common choice of treatment and patients were locked up, never to be seen again. But in these enlightened times, treatment for the mentally ill is frequently confusing, fragmented, frustrating, and often geared for certain social classes rather than the masses. All is cause for a lot of concern and anguish to victim and family when time of need comes around.

COMMUNITY MENTAL HEALTH

For close to 200 years the mental hospital was the primary place for the care and treatment of patients with serious psychological disorders. But in the past 20 years a lot of changes have been made. The mental hospital is becoming a thing of the past. In 1955 only 23 percent of psychiatric patients were treated in outpatient facilities—the remaining 77 percent were in either mental hospitals or psychiatric units of general hospitals. By 1977 the figures were almost reversed—76 percent of psychiatric patients received care in outpatient or community mental health centers, while 24 percent received hospital care. The trend to deinstitutionalize mental patients and look for support from community health agencies continues to grow and affect all aspects of psychiatric care.

When community mental health centers started up 20 years ago, there were approximately 700 located in different parts of the country. These programs were funded by the federal government but were operated by state and local groups and agencies. While the idea was good, insufficient funding kept hundreds more from ever being established.

Today there is no clear definition of what constitutes a community mental health center—some offer only outpatient services and some provide a comprehensive program including outpatient, inpatient, and after care. At all centers, services are paid for on a sliding scale, according to ability to pay.

If a patient or family member called the San Diego County Mental Health Service, for example, he or she would be referred to a counselor who would either answer specific questions about services, set up an appointment within a reasonable time, or have the patient seen immediately. If necessary, a patient could be admitted to the inpatient unit for observation and/or treatment. What San Diego offers, however, is probably not the same as what your community offers. And, most likely, what your community offers is different from what you'll find across the county line. The only way to find out what services are available is to call your local mental health association and ask. And it might be best to find out what's out there *before* the need should ever arise.

THE WARNING SIGNS OF TROUBLE

Which brings us to the question: How *do* you know when it's time to seek help for emotional troubles? The National Institute of Mental Health says there are five warning signals that can sometimes help to identify someone who needs help (especially if these signals continue for any length of time).

- Is this person acting differently than he usually does? Can you link this change in behavior to something that has happened recently? Any event such as the death of a close relative, or even something positive—like a job promotion—can trigger a troublesome emotional reaction.

- Does the individual seem to be excessively withdrawn and depressed? Are hobbies, friends, and relatives ignored suddenly? Is there a feeling that this person has begun to lose confidence in himself or herself? Depressive illnesses have many symptoms similar to these.
- Does the person complain of episodes of extreme, almost uncontrollable, anxiety? Is this anxiety unrelated to any normal concern, such as a child's illness or a backlog of bills? Anxiety that has no discernible cause is a sign of an emotional difficulty.
- Does the individual become aggressive, rude, and abusive over minor incidents? Are there remarks about groups or individuals "out to get him"? If that last remark was made in all seriousness, and blowups and violent physical behavior occur, there is a strong indication some help may be required.
- Is there a change in the person's habits, such as eating, sleeping, or grooming? Suddenly, has the individual almost stopped eating? Conversely, has he or she started eating or drinking a lot in a compulsive manner? Either sleeplessness or too much sleeping can be an indicator.

If you answer yes to any one of these questions, you could need help. I'd suggest your first step is to see a therapist.

HOW TO FIND A THERAPIST

If your emotional problems are sufficiently incapacitating that you can no longer handle them alone, don't be ashamed to seek help from a licensed therapist. A visit with a therapist does not mean that you're a "weak" person or, worse, that your life and emotions are out of control. It does mean that you recognize you have a problem and are turning to a professional to get it "fixed" (in the same way that you would turn to an orthopedist if you broke your leg).

There are many different kinds of therapists qualified to give counseling. Which one you choose often depends on the nature of the problem and its severity. Following is a listing of mental health professionals, and a description of what each does.

Pastoral Counselor—Most pastors who have special training in psychology or social work or have degrees in these fields can provide helpful, inexpensive counseling. In most cases a pastor is not a member of the psychiatric team, so he should be willing to refer patients to an appropriate professional therapist if necessary.

Psychologist—This person holds a degree in psychology, which is the study of the human mind and human behavior. A clinical psychologist has a doctoral degree in psychology plus a year of supervised clinical training and successful completion of a state licensing examination.

The cost of therapy provided by a clinical psychologist is reimbursed under most medical insurance policies, as is the more traditional care offered by a psychiatrist. A psychologist frequently charges less than a psychiatrist and can be just as effective. The psychologist should have a license and should be certified by the American Board of Examiners in Professional Psychology.

Psychiatric-Mental Health Nurse—This therapist is an RN with additional education (usually a master's degree in the field). Psychiatric nurses specialize in the prevention, treatment, and rehabilitation of mental illness. They conduct individual, family, and group therapy.

Psychiatric Social Worker—This individual has advanced training in social work with a specialty in psychiatry. Most psychiatric social workers have a master's degree and usually work in hospitals or community health centers.

Psychiatrist—This is a medical doctor who specializes in the treatment of mental illness. A psychiatrist must complete a medical degree, then after a year of internship, complete a three-year residency in psychiatry. A psychiatrist can prescribe drugs, while other therapists may recommend that their client's physician write a prescription. A psychiatrist should have a state license and should be certified by the American Board of Psychiatry and Neurology.

Psychoanalyst—Generally, this is a psychiatrist with special training in the use of psychoanalysis as a treatment method. There are also lay analysts who treat patients by psychoanalysis but who are not psychiatrists.

Psychotherapists—This is a generic term for any one of the above professionally trained persons who treat mental illness or personality disorders by psychological means.

If you doubt the credentials of any therapist, check with the local department of mental health or the individual professional association.

Perhaps the easiest and most common way to find a qualified therapist is to contact the nearest community mental health center (if it's not listed that way in the telephone book, look under "Hospitals," "Clinics," or "Physicians" in the Yellow Pages).

The Rules of the Game

Once you've begun therapy and have established a satisfactory relationship with a therapist, you should follow the doctor's or therapist's orders (according to one psychiatric nurse, for example, manic depressive and schizophrenic patients sometimes stop taking medication when they begin to feel better. As a result, they often end up getting sick and have to return to the hospital).

Regardless of a therapist's credentials, be wary of those who try such treatments as massage, manipulation, or strange diets to cure mental ills. *Immediately* leave a therapist who suggests a sexual relationship as part of therapy. The American Psychiatric Association and the American Medical Association are strongly opposed to this type of "treatment."

If the therapy or therapist isn't working out, try to find out why by first speaking with the therapist. If the discussion is unsatisfactory, you can get a second opinion, change therapists, change therapy programs, or even discontinue treatment altogether. (You should, however, be fully informed of the implications of completely discontinuing treatment.)

HOW TO GET HELP IN A HURRY

Sometimes an emotionally ill person can't wait for the "next available appointment." If a troubled individual becomes violent, gets completely out of control, or tries to commit suicide, where do you turn for help?

If the patient is already in therapy, contact the therapist for advice.

If you have no therapist but have a family physician, call this person. He may see the patient right away, refer him to a therapist, or send him directly to the hospital emergency room—whichever is most appropriate. Your family physician may suggest you call an ambulance to transport the patient to the hospital. Look in the Yellow Pages under "Ambulances" or call the police, fire department, or rescue squad if any of these provide ambulance service in your community.

Contact the nearest community mental health center for advice. If it's an emergency, contact the suicide prevention center, drug hot line or mental health hot line. If you're unable to find the number for these services in the front of your phone book, ask the operator for assistance.

In a crisis situation or if there is a strong possibility that the person may injure himself or others, call the police.

WHEN HOSPITALIZATION IS NECESSARY

Sometimes it's obvious that there's no choice. In the best interests of the patient and/or his family, short-term hospitalization may be the only possible treatment. But how do you know what facilities are available and which one is best? To be honest, you will not have to run from place to place to select a facility, because there aren't that many available.

There are three basic types of facilities where psychiatric care is provided: a public institution (state mental health hospitals or inpatient community center, if available), a private facility, and a psychiatric unit in a general hospital.

State-run institutions now admit only a small number of patients and usually only admit them after they've been evaluated in another facility. In California, for example, there are 5,000 beds in state mental hospitals (ten years ago there were 30,000 to 40,000 beds). Of the present 5,000 beds, about half are occupied by the criminally insane or sex offenders, who by law must be confined. The remainder of the patients are the demented elderly with a diagnosis of schizophrenia or an affective disorder, such as manic-depression. California is not alone in its reluctance to admit new patients into state mental hospitals.

Deinstitutionalization officially began in 1963 when Congress passed the Community Mental Health Centers Act. This law required the development of a network of mental health centers that would provide comprehensive care to the mentally ill. Thus were born the community health programs. Deinstitutionalization came about because many felt that mental hospitals were antitherapeutic and that the legal rights of mental patients were violated when they were committed to hospitals involuntarily. Many experts believe that deinstitutionalization would have been impossible if antipsychotic drugs had not been developed in the 1950s and 1960s. By controlling the severity of patients' symptoms, the emotionally ill would be better able to participate in community-based programs.

As part of the community health center system, patients may be able to receive short-term hospital care in the community. But care in these facilities is variable. For those who are able to pay, the preferred option is often a private psychiatric hospital or a psychiatric unit in a general hospital. Which is best?

Selecting a psychiatric facility depends on the nature of the patient's problem, what kind of therapy is indicated, and how much money the family has to spend (insurance coverage for psychiatric problems varies with different plans and policies—most of the time it's not enough).

The trend in most hospitals today is toward early discharge for the mentally ill patient, so regardless of the facility selected, the stay will be counted in days or weeks rather than months or years.

For most psychiatric problems that require short-term care, a small unit in a general hospital may be adequate. But if a patient is in need of a special program, he is not apt to find it in a small facility. For the safety of the patient and to insure that the greatest progress can be made, a patient should be in a unit with patients who have a similar diagnosis and are at a similar level of incapacity. A paranoid schizophrenic who suffers from delusions, for example, should not room with a patient who suffers from severe depression. In a large facility, this is not likely to happen. In a small unit, it could.

Evaluating the Facility

One of the first questions you should ask in any facility is: What kind of therapy is offered and who gets this therapy? Is the hospital flexible in its approach to treatment? If one particular therapy is *never* done or is *always* done, you should be suspicious, since the best therapy is the one that is tailored to the individual patient. Psychiatry is an inexact science, and in the best interests of the patient, there should be a variety of options in therapy and in therapists. In most hospitals, psychiatrists prescribe medications, but psychologists, psychiatric social workers, psychiatric nurses, aides, occupational and recreational therapists, and others carry out the program.

A patient can receive early emergency care in a psychiatric unit in a general hospital while family members investigate the options available. When visiting a facility, make a list of the questions that are important to you. Ask the director, psychiatrist, or social worker about cost, therapy, the usual routine of the facility, when the patient can be allowed to have visitors, and when he can leave the grounds on a "pass." Once the patient is admitted, you should know whom to contact about the patient's progress—what's the telephone number and the best time of day to call?

After the Stay Is Over

Following discharge from a psychiatric hospital, there should be some place where a patient can continue to receive guidance, support, and care. Unfortunately, the supply of facilities does not begin to meet the need.

If it's possible, home care—living with family members or in a loving foster home—is the best solution *for the patient*. Unfortunately, it's not always the best solution for the family. In many cases home care is not possible because families don't have the assistance of therapists or self-help groups to give direction and to relieve caretakers of some of the tremendous responsibilities that are placed on their shoulders.

If home care is not possible, another option is a halfway house. Usually state supported, halfway houses have a live-in couple who acts as managers or "houseparents." In the best of situations, the residents of halfway houses act as members of a large extended family (a halfway house generally houses 10 to 20 ex-patients). The managers and other counselors help residents to find some type of employment and to learn the social skills that are necessary for survival. As residents prepare to move out (usually after six months) they spend less and less time in the house, only the evenings and weekends, while their days are occupied with school, a job, volunteer work, or employment in a sheltered workshop.

There are some halfway houses in this country that stand as shining examples of what can be accomplished. But there are too few (less than 1,000 in the whole country). One of the main reasons for the lack of halfway houses is that many people don't want them located in their neighborhoods.

Some states have developed a system of board and care homes that offer a more permanent solution for former patients. These facilities are usually privately run but are licensed by the state. Each needs to be evaluated individually.

For many psychiatric patients who are elderly or chronically ill, the only option is placement in a nursing home. (It's estimated that 75 percent of the men and women over 65 years of age who now reside in nursing homes have mental disorders.) In some cases nursing homes are more degrading and inhumane than the old mental hospitals. Some families, however, may have no alternative but to place a loved one in a nursing home. If such a move is necessary, the family should select a home carefully and visit it often to monitor the kind of care that is given.

KEEPING YOURSELF EMOTIONALLY FIT

None of us can pick our parents or our genetic makeup, but as adults we do have a certain amount of control over our lives. A balanced diet and regular exercise are important factors in maintaining emotional as well as physical health. Having a good family life and friendships with good, positive people is also important in keeping a person mentally alert and emotionally strong. Talking over your troubles with a trusted friend, expressing your emotions in a diary, or praying away your troubles are all methods that have been used successfully by emotionally troubled (especially depressed) individuals.

It is not always possible or necessary to seek professional guidance every time a personal problem arises. Severity and duration of symptoms are two of the most important criteria when deciding if outside help is needed.

On a day-to-day basis, it's most important to know how to resolve normal conflicts and issues at the time they occur. This learned skill improves with maturity. Some people speed up this process by attending seminars or reading popular books on the subject of emotional health. Some of these seminars and books are worthwhile—many are not. To avoid throwing money away and possibly increasing your emotional turmoil, I would suggest carefully examining the credentials of any person who is in charge of a group program. Be skeptical. Beware of trendy therapies that are here today and will be gone tomorrow.

For the novice reader, the most comprehensive books on emotional health and various therapies are probably beginning-level psychology textbooks. University libraries and bookstores as well as community bookstores would have these on hand. Read the most recent text you can find for an overview of the subject.

In addition, a large number of mass-market publications can be useful in working on issues that cause personal and social discomfort. And don't overlook the many religious books on the market that have proved to be helpful in handling some of life's problems.

Finally, always consider the possibility that your or another's symptoms of distress may be caused by a physical rather than an emotional problem. Anxiety, for example, can result from a psychological dilemma or it can be caused by an overactive thyroid or low blood sugar.

Consider also the dreaded diagnosis of Alzheimer's disease. This malady, the most common form of dementia, causes intellectual deterioration, disorganization of personality, and inability to carry out the normal tasks of daily living. But dementia also can be caused by drug intoxication, depression, head injuries, brain tumors, and nutritional deficiencies such as pernicious anemia.

It's important, therefore, that a thorough medical screening be carried out on all emotionally ill patients before a diagnosis is made and a course of treatment prescribed.

Chapter 11

HOSPITALIZATION— THE INSIDE STORY

Chances are that if you've never worked in a hospital or been a patient in a hospital, you think that one is as good (or as bad) as another. But is fast food the same as French cuisine? Is a DC-3 the same as a 747? Of course not. Here's what you should know if your *only* choice is to go to the hospital.

ALL HOSPITALS ARE NOT THE SAME

It is true that all of the 7,000 hospitals in the United States provide care for the sick and injured. But there's significant variation in how these medical services are provided.

For example, hospitals can be large (500 beds or more); average sized (200 to 500 beds); or small (fewer than 200 beds). Hospitals can be short term (average stay of less than 30 days) or long term (stay is greater than 30 days). Most hospitals in this country care for patients with a wide variety of ailments and are referred to as a general hospital (as in the soap opera of the same name). But there are a substantial number of specialized hospitals that treat only cancer patients or psychiatric patients or those requiring rehabilitation (to name a few).

Finally, hospitals can be classified according to ownership. There are private hospitals, some run for profit, some not for profit, and there are public hospitals that may or may not be connected with a university but are supported by local, state, or federal tax money.

In recent years, increasing numbers of profit-making hospitals have opened their doors. Of the 7,000 hospitals in this country, 1,003 are now classified as "investor owned" or independently owned and are run for profit. The largest of these investor-owned hospital chains is the Hospital Corporation of America with 202 hospitals; Humana Inc. with 88; and American Medical International with 73. Humana of Louisville, Kentucky, is the facility where William Schroeder received his artificial heart. Humana is representative of the new investor-owned companies that are providing money-saving and efficient methods. They are challenging community hospitals and nonprofit organizations for a greater share of the nearly $1-billion-a-day health care industry.

What is the reputation of these new profit-making hospitals? *The New England Journal of Medicine* recently published a study suggesting that some California investor-owned hospitals charge more than the nonprofit hospitals but do not offer any better care or service. However, there are some who cast a jaundiced eye on such studies. They feel that profit-making hospitals do not charge more but are a threat to doctors and nonprofit hospitals. Supporters feel that profit-making hospitals are a good prescription for the ailing health care industry.

If you're going to be a patient in a hospital, it's not that important whether the institution you're considering is investor owned or supported by tax money. What *is* important is how appropriate the hospital is for your particular medical problem and how well the hospital is run.

WHICH HOSPITAL'S FOR YOU?

To begin with, you should know the basic differences between a medical center hospital and a community hospital. The former is larger and is usually connected with a medical school. Medical center hospitals also have house staffs (interns and residents who are present 24 hours a day) and separate departments (medicine, surgery, pediatrics, and so on) that are headed by full-time physicians who teach and supervise the medical care in their particular department. Besides caring for patients, medical centers train future doctors as well as nurses and other personnel (and so are called "teaching hospitals"). Medical centers also carry out research. Sometimes priorities get mixed up in this system, and what is in the best interests of education or research may not be in the best interests of the patient.

And now community hospitals. These *can* be teaching hospitals and they *can* have house staffs and department heads but usually they don't. Community hospitals usually exist for the sole purpose of providing medical care to members of the community.

So now you're going to be a patient in the hospital. Do you choose a medical center hospital or a community hospital?

Medical Center Hospitals

If you have a complicated medical problem or have suffered severe burns or need brain surgery or a kidney transplant (to name a few serious and complex conditions), you would probably receive the best care in a medical center. These institutions are top of the line for medical diagnosis and treatment because they have the latest equipment and the most experienced physicians. Should an emergency arise any time of the day or night, competent care is only a few moments away.

But medical center institutions are apt to be impersonal, chaotic, and more interested in you as a subject for medical study than you as a person. The politics of care in a medical center hospital are very different from the politics of any other organization on the "outside." If you're a bank president with hemorrhoids, for example, you won't get as much attention from the staff as the derelict in the next bed who suffers from lupus erythematosus. In a teaching hospital, it's not who you are that counts, it's what you have.

A frequent complaint of patients in medical center hospitals is the constant coming and going of personnel. Patients are questioned and examined time and again. This can be inconvenient and tiring.

Community Hospitals

Community hospitals offer less fragmented and more personalized care to their patients. In a good community hospital the nursing staff is more likely to see you as a person rather than an interesting case. Staff members may be more kind to family members too, and may "bend the rules" to accommodate unusual circumstances. Because your personal physician is *the* physician in charge of your care, you are less apt to receive conflicting advice and are more likely to be able to participate in decisions regarding your care.

However, if you're a patient in a community hospital that has no house staff, and an emergency arises, you may have to wait for your physician to drive across town to attend to your needs. If you have a serious medical problem, like heart disease, this could jeopardize your care. If you have surgery in a community hospital, you may be "put under" by a nurse anesthetist rather than a board-certified anesthesiologist. This may not be in your best interests. And finally, if you're having surgery that is even moderately complex, the surgeon who operates out of a community hospital may not have the necessary experience and up-to-date techniques (as well as the latest equipment) that will assure the best surgical outcome for you.

So again, your selection of a hospital depends on what your medical problem is. If it falls into the "serious" category (complex medical problems or sophisticated diagnostic studies; major trauma or extensive surgical procedures like open heart surgery), your best bet is a medical center. If your problem falls into the "routine" category (simple tests, uncomplicated medical problems), the community hospital will serve your needs adequately. The mid-level problems are the surgeries that require general anesthesia but are not major procedures, and also some medical emergencies such as heart attack, stroke, or severe asthma. The deciding factor in selecting a medical center hospital or community hospital for these mid-level problems is the quality of care that you'll receive at the particular hospital.

DETERMINING QUALITY OF CARE

The first thing you should check is accreditation. Hospitals are accredited by individual states and by the Joint Commission on Accreditation of Hospitals (JCAH). The JCAH, sponsored by the American College of Physicians, the American College of Surgeons, the American Hospital Association, and the American Medical Association, is neither a profit-making nor a government institution. Accreditation by this group is voluntary. However, it is often required by third-party payers such as Medicare, Medicaid, and private insurance plans. The fact that a hospital is accredited by the JCAH generally means that its facility is safe and has met established standards for operation.

Over half the hospitals in this country are accredited by the JCAH. Most accredited hospitals will display their JCAH certificates prominently in the lobby. You can contact the local county medical society to find out if the hospital you're considering is accredited. If it's not accredited, you might want to find out why it isn't before automatically dismissing the hospital as second rate.

What's Its Reputation?

Paramedics are excellent resource people when it comes to which hospital is best for emergency problems. They know which hospitals have doctors on call 24 hours a day and which one they'd want to be taken to if necessary.

Nurses generally know which hospitals give the best nursing care. They know which ones have the highest nurse-to-patient ratio; which have the lowest turnover of nurses; and which are staffed by full-time versus part-time or agency nurses. High nurse-to-patient ratio and continuity of nursing care are significant factors in determining the quality of care you will receive in any hospital. If you know several nurses, ask their opinions about the hospitals in your community.

Physicians will generally become patients at hospitals where they feel that the best physicians are attending or are on staff. They may select a surgeon because he has privileges at a particular hospital or because he works with a particular anesthesiologist. So ask your physician or a physician-friend which hospital he would choose if he or a member of his family had a medical problem like yours.

THE BOTTOM LINE—GOING WHERE YOUR PHYSICIAN HAS "PRIVILEGES"

If you've had some experience as a hospital patient, you may think that all this discussion of "choosing" a hospital is academic. Suppose, for example, you're 200 miles from home and you have a heart attack or are involved in a serious automobile accident. You will obviously go to whichever hospital the ambulance takes you to and pray you will be in good hands.

But even when you're close to home and your hospital trip is more or less "planned," you may feel you have no choice because everyone knows that a patient goes to the hospital where his doctor has privileges. Right? Not necessarily.

First, what is meant by "hospital privileges?" Hospitals have medical boards that determine which physicians can be "attending" and which can have the privilege of admitting patients. If your doctor does not have privileges at a certain hospital, you cannot be a patient in that hospital unless you want to change doctors. Some physicians have privileges or are "attendings" at several hospitals, in which case you may have a choice as to where you go.

Usually, if you live in a small to moderate-sized community and your medical problem is fairly routine, you will go to the hospital where your physician has privileges. It's easier that way—you have continuity of care and it's convenient for you and your family.

But suppose you're new in town and don't have a primary care physician? Or suppose you feel that your problem necessitates a more sophisticated approach than the community hospital can offer? Or suppose, after checking out your community hospital, you find that it offers substandard care, while the hospital in the next town has an excellent reputation? In any of these cases, it's *your* privilege to choose the hospital that you want (assuming of course that you have the time and resources to make such a choice). You may have to temporarily change doctors or you may have to travel out of town or even out of state, but it is *your* choice and there's no one who will consider all the alternatives as carefully as you.

IF THE PATIENT IS A CHILD

Books have been written on the subject of hospitalization of children. The essence of the messages in these books is as follows:

- Hospitalization can be a scary experience for a young child and should be avoided whenever possible. Get a second opinion, consider alternative treatments or outpatient care. Hospitalization is definitely a last resort. In an emergency or life-threatening situation, of course, hospitalization will be the only resort.

- If you have a choice, select a hospital that specializes in treating children. Next best is a medical center with a large pediatric service. A general hospital with a "few" pediatric beds should be your last choice.
- If possible, prepare your child for hospitalization before the day of admission. Have a frank discussion with the child's doctor so that you, as an adult, will know what to expect. Then communicate this information to your child in language that is honest and straightforward. Explain what will happen in the hospital and how long the stay will be. Try to anticipate problems and misunderstandings. Accept the child's feelings of fear and anger.
- Take advantage of any preadmission preparation that the hospital offers—a walking tour of the facilities, a movie or puppet show on hospitalization. Ask questions and encourage your child to do the same.
- Stay with your child as much as possible. If the staff disapproves, insist quietly—but firmly—that you plan to stay by your child's side. Be prepared to "sleep" in a chair and be prepared to get nasty looks from the staff. No matter. Your concern is for your child's emotional and physical well-being. If push turns to shove, you can ask your physician to write an "order" that you be allowed to stay with your child.

MEETING THE ADMISSION CLERK

You decide to take your doctor's recommendation and be admitted to the hospital of your choice. One morning the admitting office calls to say there's a bed ready. They'll be expecting you between 2 and 3 P.M. the next day. (This is the usual time for admission, although some hospitals admit early in the morning to save time and money for the patients. If that sounds good to you, ask your physician if you can be admitted early in the morning.) Your bag has been packed for a week. Time hangs heavy.

The next day, you go to the admitting office, as you were told, and the clerk has many questions—mostly they concern your insurance and how you plan to pay for the hospitalization. You probably were told what information to bring in with you—the usual is your Social Security card or number; your insurance, Medicare, or Medicaid card or number; and the name, address, and phone number of your employer, your spouse, and a person to call in case of an emergency.

While in the admitting office you may be asked to sign a blanket consent form and/or release form. You may be reluctant to do this, although the clerk will probably say you can't be admitted unless the forms are signed. Don't be too concerned about the forms. Any procedures that you have done in the hospital will have to be explained to you before the procedure can be carried out (the subject of informed consent will be discussed later). In addition, your signature on any blanket form could never release the hospital from legal responsibility in case of negligence. It just wouldn't hold up in court.

You will find when you are admitted to a hospital that one of the categories that you're put under, in addition to your diagnosis ("she's a gallbladder" or "he's a low-back pain"), is whose patient you are or whose service you're on. You're the patient of whichever doctor referred you to the hospital, whether this is your primary care physician, a surgeon, pediatrician, or obstetrician. You may also be referred to as a patient on a certain service, such as the medical service, surgical service, pediatric service, and so on. This will determine which floor you will stay on. In a large teaching hospital, medical patients with different diagnoses will probably not be mixed in together but will be in separate units requiring the following specialty services:

- Cardiology (heart problems)
- Dermatology (diseases of the skin)
- Endocrinology (metabolic disorders)
- Gastroenterology (conditions of the stomach and intestine)
- Genitourinary (diseases of the male reproductive and urinary system as well as diseases of the female urinary system)
- Gynecology (diseases of the female reproductive system)
- Hematology (blood disorders)
- Nephrology (diseases of the kidney)
- Neurology (diseases of the nervous system)
- Oncology (cancer)
- Ophthalmology (diseases of the eye)
- Orthopedics (diseases of the bones and supporting structures)
- Otorhinolaryngology (disorders of the ear, nose, and throat)
- Pulmonary disease (conditions affecting the lungs)
- Rheumatology (arthritis)

If you're being admitted to a medical center (teaching) hospital and have no specific referring physician, you become a "staff patient," which means that a house staff doctor (who is on the hospital payroll) will be in charge of your care.

Once your ID bracelet has been snapped on your wrist—usually in the admitting office—you are officially "in" and you will be taken to your room. The ritual of hospitalization will begin.

SOME TIPS WORTH REMEMBERING

If it's at all possible, you should have all medical tests (x-rays, blood work, urinalysis) done prior to admission, unless the tests are very complex and are the main reason for hospitalization. If tests are completed ahead of time and if your admission physical examination is completed ahead of time, it will save you money and may save you a day or two of hospitalization. If you're having surgery, for example, you may be admitted to the hospital on the day of the operation.

Avoid being admitted on a Saturday, because most routine tests and elective surgery will not be done until Monday. Try to be discharged before the weekend too. Finally, avoid being admitted on or around a major holiday.

If you're going to be a patient in a medical center hospital, avoid being admitted on or near July 1, because this is the traditional day when new interns and residents arrive at the hospital to begin training.

A ROOM OF YOUR OWN

You should consider getting a private hospital room if:

- Being alone—having peace and quiet—is a top priority in your life.
- You don't want to be disturbed by a roommate who is seriously ill or unpleasant or one who smokes, snores, turns the TV up too loud, or has disagreeable visitors. Of course it's difficult to know ahead of time whether you'll get a good or bad roommate. Sometimes it's just the luck of the draw.
- You want to live by *your* schedule, watch the TV shows *you* like, and sleep when *you* want (just being a patient in a

hospital, of course, precludes a certain amount of independence).

- You plan to use your hospital stay to catch up on office work or personal correspondence (realistically, you probably won't feel like doing too much serious work while you're in the hospital).
- You expect a lot of visitors and don't want them inconvenienced by the presence of other patients and visitors in your room (if your social life is this important to you, you probably aren't sick enough to be in a hospital—you may be better off recuperating in a hotel).

You should consider having a roommate (or roommates) if:

- You can't afford the extra cost of a private room.
- You're a "people person" who prefers conversation rather than long quiet spells (if you're not expecting many visitors, or if your hospital stay will be long, having a roommate may be just the right prescription for combating loneliness).
- You're afraid that the nurses will "forget you" if your private room is tucked away in a distant corner (sometimes this *does* seem to be the case—nurses try to keep the sickest patients near the nurses' station so they can keep an eye on them).
- You're afraid that if you fall out of bed, slip on the floor, or suffer a heart attack, you'll be alone and unable to get help quickly (if the patient in question is elderly, confused, or unable to get about freely, having a roommate *can* be a definite asset).

To be perfectly honest, whether you have a roommate or not usually depends on two factors:

- Can you afford it? Many insurance companies won't pay the extra expense, so ask first.
- Is there a private room available?

If you've been assigned to a roommate who is less than what you expected, you might try "discussion and compromise" as a solution to your difficulties. This is probably the best alternative if your hospital stay is short. But if your roommate is making life absolutely miserable for you, and your expected stay is at least a week, you can ask to have your room changed. But don't expect the nursing staff to be excited about doing this for you. Approximately 20 departments in the hospital (from the admitting office to the kitchen, from the business office to the lab) will have to be notified if you change rooms. A room switch costs the hospital a good deal of time and money. However, if your roommate situation is hopeless, stick to your guns and insist on a room change. The $100 or so that the hospital will have to lay out to make the switch will be cost effective if it gives you peace of mind.

HOSPITAL PATIENTS DO HAVE RIGHTS

The "Hospital Patients' Bill of Rights" was published in 1973 by the American Hospital Association. A copy of this document should be conspicuously displayed in every hospital or, better yet, distributed to every patient before or at the time of hospital admission. If you've been a patient in a hospital but have never seen a copy of the bill of rights, that may tell you volumes about the hospital's attitude toward its patients.

The basic "Hospital Patients' Bill of Rights" sets a minimum standard for patients. Some feel that the document is not hard enough on hospitals and doctors and that much more should be included. But the document is at least a base line for further statements on patients' rights. Frankly, it would be nice if all hospitals followed the present guidelines.

You Call This Courteous!

Items 1, 7, 8, and 10 of the bill of rights (see pages 176–77) guarantee little more than courteous and considerate treatment of the hospitalized patient. These could be called the "golden rules" of hospital care (doing to others as we would have them do to us). In many hospitals the simple courtesies of life are violated time and again:

- Doctors discuss your case as though you were not present.
- Personnel refer to you by your first name (even though you're old enough to be their parent).
- Nurses awaken you during the night to give you a sleeping pill.
- Curtains are not drawn when you're given a bedpan.

HOSPITAL PATIENTS' BILL OF RIGHTS

1. The patient has the right to considerate and respectful care by competent personnel.

2. The patient has the right to obtain from his physician complete current information concerning his diagnosis, treatment, and prognosis in terms the patient can be reasonably expected to understand. When it is not medically advisable to give such information to the patient, the information should be made available to an appropriate person in his behalf. He has the right to know, by name, the physician responsible for coordinating his care.

3. The patient has the right to receive from his physician information necessary to give informed consent prior to the start of any procedure and/or treatment. Except in emergencies, such information for informed consent should include, but not necessarily be limited to, the specific procedure and/or treatment, the medically significant risks involved, and the probable duration of incapacitation. Where medically significant alternatives for care or treatment exist, or when the patient requests information concerning medical alternatives, the patient has the right to such information. The patient also has the right to know the name of the person responsible for the procedures and/or treatment.

4. The patient has the right to refuse treatment to the extent permitted by law, and to be informed of the medical consequences of his action.

5. The patient has the right to every consideration of privacy concerning his own medical care program. Case discussion, consultation, examination, and treatment are confidential and should be conducted discreetly. Those not directly involved in his care must have the permission of the patient to be present.

Northwestern Memorial Hospital in Chicago recently sponsored a five-hour mandatory seminar for employees on "niceness." This was done after a patient survey revealed that hospital care was "too impersonal." Almost all of the hospital employees attended the seminar and improved their "niceness quotient." However, only one of five doctors signed up for the course. Apparently they didn't feel the need to improve their behavior.

If you're a hospital patient and you feel that you've been treated discourteously, what should you do? You can speak to the discourteous person yourself, although that's a hard thing to do if you're feeling rotten (and presumably you're feeling rotten or you wouldn't be in a hospital). In some cases it's better if you have a family

6. The patient has the right to expect that all communications and records pertaining to his care will be treated as confidential.

7. The patient has the right to expect that within its capacity a hospital must make reasonable response to the request of a patient for services. The hospital must provide evaluation, service, and/or referral as indicated by the urgency of the case. When medically permissible, a patient may be transferred to another facility only after he has received complete information and explanation concerning the need for and alternatives to such a transfer. The institution to which the patient is to be transferred must first have accepted the patient for transfer.

8. The patient has the right to obtain information as to any relationship of his hospital to other health care and educational institutions insofar as his care is concerned. The patient has the right to obtain information as to the existence of any professional relationships among individuals, by name, who are treating him.

9. The patient has the right to be advised if the hospital proposes to engage in or perform human experimentation affecting his care or treatment. The patient has the right to refuse to participate in such research projects.

10. The patient has the right to expect reasonable continuity of care. He has the right to know in advance what appointment times and physicians are available and where. The patient has the right to expect that the hospital will provide a mechanism whereby he is informed by his physician or a delegate of the physician of the patient's continuing health.

spokesman or an advocate speak to the discourteous employee. If speaking directly to the person doesn't help, you or your advocate can report the incident to the patient representative or ombudsman (most hospitals now have at least one on staff).

Confidentiality—It Should Be a "Given"

Items 5 and 6 of the patients' bill of rights deal with confidentiality, which has always been considered the cornerstone of the doctor-patient relationship. But things are more complicated now than they were during the time of Hippocrates. In even an average-sized hospital, many different health workers can have access to your medical records. In a teaching hospital especially, many different people may want to watch your surgery, examine your body, or discuss your case. Some of this is to your advantage—several heads may be better than one when it comes to making a definitive diagnosis or determining the proper mode of treatment.

To be perfectly honest, once you step into a hospital, privacy goes out the window. But a patient is not totally helpless. If, for example, you don't want a gaggle of young medical students looking on while your physician does a proctoscopic exam, you have the legal right to refuse their admittance to the procedure. And if there's some bit of information that you don't want included in your hospital record (you have a criminal record or you and your spouse are getting divorced), discuss this with your doctor before you enter the hospital. Almost all doctors will respect these special reasons for strict confidentiality.

Informed Consent— Getting the Facts and Giving Permission

Items 2, 3, 4, and 9 deal with the legal matter of informed consent.

Informed consent does not mean just signing a form that allows the doctor and hospital to "do with you what they will." It means that your doctor has spent time discussing the recommended procedure—the advantages and disadvantages, the risks, the benefits, and the alternatives. Only after this has been done and you have spent some time deciding if the recommended course of action would be in *your* best interests—only then should you consent or give permission. And if you change your mind an hour later or a week later, you have every right to rescind your permission. That's what informed consent is all about.

The late Jory Graham, a well-known journalist and advocate for cancer patients, explained her feelings on informed consent in her book *In the Company of Others:*

"As a doctrine and as a practical reality, informed consent is neither so complicated nor so difficult as doctors and lawyers would make it, nor is there any good reason for the extended medical debates it engenders. At its core, it is respect for a patient as an individual, not a defense against the possibility of a later malpractice suit."

The big problem here is that patients are not adequately informed. Most doctors are poor communicators. They speak in medical gibberish and they always leave the impression of having "better things to do" than listen and explain procedures to patients. In a recent study reported in the *Journal of the American Medical Association (JAMA)*, it was found that doctors spend very little time giving information to their patients. In recorded encounters with patients, doctors spent, on the average, a little more than a minute of explanation time in visits lasting about 20 minutes. Following these recorded meetings, the investigators asked the doctors how much time they thought they devoted to giving information. This perception was compared with the actual time measured in tape recordings. Doctors *thought* that they spent much more time informing their patients than they actually did—on the average, the doctors overestimated the time they spent giving information by about a factor of nine.

Additionally, this study showed that doctors spend more time talking with women than men, gave more information to patients who are college educated than persons who did not go to college, and explained more to patients from upper- or upper-middle-class positions than lower-class positions. Some other findings—the more uncertain a doctor was about a patient's diagnosis and prognosis, the more the doctor talked. Patients with fatal diseases, however, most frequently had information withheld from them.

In regard to doctors' characteristics and effect on communication, it was found that physicians from upper- or upper-middle-class backgrounds tended to spend more time informing their patients than doctors from lower-middle or lower-class backgrounds did. Additionally, doctors who earned less money and saw fewer patients spent more time giving out information.

Doctors are authoritarian figures. They maintain a style of high control, which is demonstrated by the fact that the vast majority of questions in a doctor-patient relationship are initiated by the doctor. The style of high control is also demonstrated by doctors frequently interrupting patients and disregarding the everyday concerns of patients.

The study reported in *JAMA* concluded: "Training programs and standards of clinical practice should emphasize that improved doctor-patient communication is both desirable and possible." Indeed.

But what if you're a patient and you don't feel that your doctor explains things to you or is withholding facts or is coercing you into treatment that is not necessary? If a specialist doesn't give you satisfactory explanations, it might be best to talk things over with your primary care physician. Or you can try asking your primary care nurse for explanations. In a teaching hospital, interns and residents can often give satisfactory explanations because they're still learning themselves. In some hospitals there are patient educators on staff— these people provide information about medical and hospital procedures.

Remember: It's your *legal* right to receive adequate explanations of all procedures that are performed in your behalf. A physician or qualified person should answer all your questions before you come to a decision. And should you change your mind *at any time,* consent for a procedure may be withdrawn.

A MATTER OF RECORDS

As soon as you are admitted to a hospital floor, there are certain SOPs (standard operating procedures) that are set into motion. One of these is putting your chart together. The chart, which hangs in a rack in the nurses' station, contains doctors' orders and progress notes, laboratory and x-ray results, medication sheet (dosage and time of administration), history and physical notes, consultation notes, surgery notes (if applicable), nursing care plans and progress notes, and additional forms and information as needed.

Patients often fear that these records contain all sorts of sensitive information concerning their personality and prognosis. Part of the reason for this fear is that patients are generally not allowed to see their charts (although almost everyone else in the hospital is allowed the privilege). And that's not fair.

If you're a patient in a hospital and you want to see a section of your chart, you might ask your primary care physician or primary care nurse if you can do so. They may accommodate your request. Legally, however, all medical records are the property of the hospital. Therefore, if you absolutely want to see your chart and the doctor and/or staff refuses to allow it, you will have to get a subpoena for the record in court.

Generally speaking, a patient's hospital chart is pretty dull fare. Hospital personnel are well aware that the patient's chart is a legal document, and so only that information which would be of legal significance is included. If a nurse questions a doctor's order and refuses to carry it out, for example, she would carefully note—in the record—the incident and what steps she took, since she could be held liable for such actions. I don't know of any nurse who would note in a chart that a patient was rude or pushy or a burden to the staff. That would be a reflection on the nurse's inability to understand and care for her patients. Such statements could also be libelous.

In addition to the "secret" patient chart, there is frequently a bedside chart that lists vital signs (temperature, pulse, respirations, and blood pressure), medications, intake and output, and other information. You're free to examine this. During your hospital stay, the medical staff should be keeping you informed as to laboratory and x-ray results and what orders have been written in your behalf. If your doctor does not volunteer this information, you should ask him yourself.

DON'T GO IT ALONE

If you're a knowledgeable health consumer and are in reasonable health, it's easy enough to visit a medical library or bookstore and gather information concerning diagnosis, treatment alternatives, as well as side effects of prescribed medications and other medical concerns. But when you're lying in a hospital bed in pain with tubes entering every orifice, how can you possibly be concerned with anything but survival?

If you're an expectant mother in the throes of labor, how can you possibly be thinking logically about safe alternatives when all you want is for the ordeal to be over?

If you're a young child separated from home and family and dropped into a strange hospital world, you're the most vulnerable of all.

No patient should have to go to a hospital without a spokesperson or advocate by his or her side or at least no farther than a phone call away. An advocate is a surrogate or a guardian angel who will speak in your behalf whenever you are unable to do so. Your advocate could be a spouse, lover, parent, child, sibling, or close friend. The first criterion is that it be a person who loves you enough to care what happens to you at every turn. Your advocate should also be someone who is assertive enough to speak up for your rights but not so abrasive that the entire staff is turned off by him or her. Sometimes a relative who is a nurse (and therefore not intimidated by the hospital system) is a good advocate. Certainly you should not select a person who "can't stand the sight of blood" or breaks out in hives when the word hospital is mentioned.

Sometimes a relative who is a lawyer makes an excellent patient advocate (although the patient may find that more than the usual number of tests will be ordered). Medical personnel fear lawsuits more than death and taxes.

Don't leave the selection of your advocate to the last minute. You want the person you select to be available at all times when you're in the hospital. That doesn't mean your advocate must sit by your side during an entire hospital stay (although with a young child that's not a bad idea). What it does mean is that the advocate has put aside this time to be your spokesperson. Make sure your primary care physician and the hospital know who this person is and know, at all times, how to contact him or her.

Finally, talk to your advocate before the time of hospitalization. Explain why you feel you will need assistance and what you expect him or her to do. Explain to your advocate—before you're hospitalized—what your expectations are in regard to hospital treatment, what heroic measures are palatable to you, and so on. Your advocate should know about your medical history, previous surgeries, and the name and dosage of any medications that you're taking (you can write all this information down ahead of time).

A patient advocate should not be confused with the hospital employee known as a hospital advocate, patient representative, or ombudsman. This person will try to resolve any problems you may have while you're a patient. As effectively as this person may be able to clear up a few minor problems, an ombudsman cannot speak for you during your entire hospital stay.

THE DELICATE ART OF BEING A PATIENT—A CHECKLIST FROM A NURSE'S POINT OF VIEW

You're a patient now and you wonder why certain things happen the way they do:

- Some evenings your 10 P.M. medication comes at 9:30 and other times it's 10:30.

- Your "hot" evening meal arrives—cold as ice. Fat globules permeate the roast beef, the gravy has congealed, the mashed potatoes can be cut with a knife, and the green beans are limp and lifeless.
- The aide insists on calling you Mrs. Parker even though you've told her on several occasions that your name is Palmer.
- One evening you're left on the bedpan for 15 minutes after the nurse answers your buzzer and says she'll be "right there."
- Your physician comes to visit and he seems distracted and moody. You ask for a change in your sleeping medication, but an hour later the nurse says that he wrote no new orders.

These are some frequent complaints of hospital patients and they are annoying scenes. But they are all what I would call minor problems in that they don't harm a patient's physical health or safety. But they're distressing enough to a patient who's already suffering, and some patients scream loud and long at such inequities (although the screams don't seem to change things much).

A hospital is not a hotel, and things do not always run smoothly. The thesis of this book is that, if possible, you should stay out of the hospital, and once admitted, you should try to get out as quickly as you can.

But while you're in the hospital, you may say, you'd like to make the best of a bad situation. And you may notice that some patients seem to be treated better than others, or at least they don't seem to have the same problems that others have. How come?

Be a Cooperative, Not Demanding, Patient

If you were faced with one of the disturbing scenes that I mentioned, your best response would be not to passively accept rude or inconsiderate behavior but to quietly discuss the matter with your primary care nurse, the head nurse, your primary care physician, or the hospital's patient representative. If you were not up to such a confrontation, you might ask your patient advocate to handle it. One discussion of any minor problem should be sufficient. If you're the kind of person who becomes hysterical over small problems, you're likely to get a reputation as a complainer, with the result that the nursing staff may not be very receptive to your future requests.

One nurse told me, "If a patient or his family is demanding, I'll pass that patient by when I'm making rounds. It might not be something I consciously do, but constant unpleasantness is not something I enjoy either."

That nurse may not be a Florence Nightingale but she's no Nurse Ratched *(One Flew Over the Cuckoo's Nest)* either. Nurses are human, after all, and they don't enjoy folks who are constantly complaining or who are never satisfied.

So my advice is to maybe overlook the very insignificant problems or quietly and politely complain to the appropriate person and then forget it. That's not being passive—that's being a cooperative patient. Other more obvious ways you can be a cooperative patient (and avoid a hospital stay that is plagued with catastrophes and bad experiences):

Be considerate of the staff. Don't push the buzzer for trivial things (especially if the nurses are very busy). Don't cry wolf.

Try to be polite. "Please" and "Thank you" are always appreciated. If you are inclined to give presents, the staff will usually enjoy a box of candy or a bouquet of flowers (give your gift while you're still a patient—you might as well receive some of the good feelings that such a gesture will generate). To some, giving gifts may sound like bribery. And I'm not suggesting that every patient needs to give presents in order to receive good care. I'm only suggesting that if you have the desire, most hospital workers will appreciate these gestures. Don't try to pay money to a nurse to get extra care or special treatment. It's just not done.

Try to be respectful of the staff as individuals as well as helping persons. Don't treat the nurses as servants or as deities either. Remember that most health workers want to help patients—that's why they chose their profession and spent long years in training. But there are few jobs that are more demanding and stressful than those in the health care field. This is not to excuse mistakes or bad behavior but to explain why it seems to be an occupational hazard.

Ask questions. Ask your doctor what his plan of approach is for you. What tests will be done? When? If surgery is planned, what will it involve? What will be the routine before surgery? After surgery?

Ask the nurse what your blood pressure is if you're curious. She should give you this information. Ask the medication nurse why you're getting a certain drug and what it should accomplish. Should the medicine be taken before or after meals? Does it matter if you take the pills a half hour early or a half hour late? If you're getting injections, could the same medicine be given by mouth? Most hospitals have a *Physicians' Desk Reference (PDR)* on every unit, so if the nurse can't answer your question immediately, she can look it up and tell you later.

Be intelligent about your care. If you're supposed to be in x-ray on Tuesday morning but no one has taken you there and it's 9 A.M. Tuesday, find out what's going on.

If the doctor prescribed a low-salt diet but you notice that your lunch tray looks exactly the same as the one for the patient in the next bed (who's on a regular diet), say something.

If a medical student comes in your room and starts to set up equipment for a blood transfusion and you haven't been told anything about it, don't let the transfusion begin until you get an explanation from the doctor in charge.

If you've always gotten two brown pills and one pink pill at 10 A.M. and one day the nurse brings you three white pills, don't take them until you make sure the new medicine is meant for you.

If your surgery is to be on your left leg and the orderly is scrubbing down your right leg, say something.

Another tip: Before you go to surgery or have any other procedure done where you'll be "out," check to make sure your identification bracelet is intact and correct. Also, if someone comes to get you for surgery and they call you Mrs. Robinson (your name is Mrs. Bertram), don't just lie there, speak up!

Find out why things happen the way they do. You may imagine one morning that the nursing staff was having quite a celebration the night before with all the noise and commotion that was going on. What may have been happening was that a seriously ill patient was admitted during the night and a large number of personnel and equipment was needed to give care. You can probably find out this information via the hospital grapevine. There's nothing wrong with that.

You may wonder too why the nurses are always late in answering your call light from 3 to 3:30 every afternoon. Change-of-shift times (7-3-11 or 8-4-12) are when almost all the nurses are tied up with patient progress reports or other duties. Try to plan ahead for requests so that you won't need assistance at these times.

Try to do as much for yourself as you are physically able to do. When the doctor says you can get up, make a real effort to do more and more for yourself. The staff will be impressed with your desire to get better and return to normal activities. It will also speed your recovery and make you feel less like a dependent patient. Of course if you're recovering from a heart attack or major surgery where absolute bed rest is required for healing, then bed rest is what it has to be.

Be a Participant in Your Care—Not a Bystander

If you're receiving intravenous (IV) therapy while in the hospital, you can handle the situation in one of several ways. You can completely let the nurses manage the IV treatment, and if they slip up and don't check and the IV becomes infiltrated (the needle gets dislodged from the vein and the fluid goes into the surrounding tissue causing pain, swelling, warmth, and redness), you can chalk up the whole experience to bad luck. Or you can get angry with the nurses and doctors and pull out the needle when you've decided you've had enough.

Another option is to become involved in the treatment and try to minimize complications. For example, ask the nurse how many drips per minute the IV is to run and what you should do if that number changes. How low should the bottle go before you call for her?

Pain control is another area where patients often suffer in silence. But you will get no gold star for being a martyr to pain. So speak up to the nurse or doctor and *demand* that changes be made if your pain medication is not doing the job. Don't wait until the middle of the night to make changes—you or your patient advocate should try to get a satisfactory order during the day shift.

The worst part of getting pain relief is waiting for the nurse to bring the medication. When you're suffering, 15 minutes can seem like an eternity. (Some nurses deliberately delay giving narcotic medication because they're afraid a patient will become addicted. For the terminally ill patient this is especially ludicrous.)

Questioning the Routines

If you've been in the hospital for a week and the nurses are still waking you up at midnight to take your vital signs, you should ask your doctor if this routine chore can be eliminated so you can get more rest.

There are many routines in hospitals that make little sense. Admission chest x-rays, for example, are standard practice in many hospitals. The custom costs as much as $1.5 billion a year, although the x-rays are usually unnecessary and fail to uncover any medical problems that would have gone undetected. And of course all x-rays pose a radiation hazard that everyone can do without. So if you're about to be admitted and the hospital wants to do a routine chest x-ray, ask your doctor if he can excuse you from having it done.

There are certain admission laboratory tests that are done "routinely" too but are of little value in detecting unknown maladies. A study reported in the *Journal of the American Medical Association* substantiates this fact.

The University of California at San Francisco medical center has approximately 8,600 elective surgical admissions per year. Certain tests, such as a complete blood cell count, are routinely done on these patients at the time of admission. The study found that 60 percent of those routinely ordered tests were not needed. The study also found that routine preoperative laboratory tests contribute little to patient care and can be eliminated without significant adverse medical consequences.

So what should all this mean to you? It means that if your scheduled hospital visit is for elective surgery, check with your surgeon about the necessity of having blood drawn for "routine" admission tests. If the tests are not necessary, why should you go through the expense and bother of having them done?

Of course you can't question everything that goes on in the hospital, but if something seems off-base to you, check it out and see if you can skip it. Just because a hospital practice is routine doesn't make it right or mean that it's in your best interests.

Sound Off!

If, in spite of your best efforts, a serious hospital problem arises (you receive the wrong dosage of medicine and suffer a reaction or no nurse answers your call light and you fall in the bathroom), you should bring out the big guns and scream loud and clear. If you're uncertain whom to complain to, the chart on page 188 may help.

Of course the ultimate complaint is leaving the hospital against medical advice (AMA)—or going AWOL.

If you've decided to cancel the surgery or decided you've had enough of the hospital's pills and potions, nobody can keep you against your will. If the doctor wants you to stay, you can still leave but will have to sign yourself out "AMA." This is how the incident will be written on your chart (to protect the doctor and hospital in case of a lawsuit).

HOW TO LODGE A COMPLAINT

Nature of Problem	*Direct Complaints To:*
Problems with nursing staff	First talk to the primary care nurse (if you have one), then head nurse. If they don't give you satisfaction, report to supervisor and finally nursing director.
Problems with medical staff (interns, residents, medical students, consultants)	First talk to primary care or attending physician, then direct complaint to chief of particular service (medicine, surgery) and finally to medical director.
Problems with food	Contact dietician (if you don't know how to contact her, ask head nurse).
Hospital is dirty or repairs are needed	Talk to head nurse or contact housekeeping department directly. If not satisfactory, contact administrator.
Problems with bill	Contact business office.

As a free citizen, you're perfectly within your rights to leave the hospital this way. And it will not jeopardize your chances of being readmitted to the hospital later. Just be sure, before signing yourself out, that you know what your medical options are and check with your insurance company to be sure they will still cover your bill.

Chapter *12*

STAYING WELL

If I told you I had a magic formula that could lengthen your life by ten years, decrease your chances of getting sick by 50 percent, and possibly keep you out of the hospital forever, would you be willing to try it? Using my formula won't cost you a penny (beginning to sound even better, isn't it?) but you may have to change the way you do a few things.

Many years ago, Lester Breslow, MD, then dean of UCLA's School of Public Health, found that certain health practices correlated with increased longevity. They became the seven cardinal rules of good living. They were:

- Get regular exercise.
- Don't smoke.
- Maintain normal weight.
- Eat breakfast.

- Avoid heavy use of alcohol.
- Sleep eight hours each night.
- Avoid snacks between meals.

A lot of time has gone by since Dr. Breslow came up with his formula. It's time for a new one. Based on the latest findings in improving longevity and quality of life, I modernized Dr. Breslow's rules and came up with a formula of my own to reflect the lifestyles of the '80s. Here, then, is my "magic formula."

- Get plenty of exercise.
- Don't smoke.
- Maintain normal weight.
- Follow a sensible diet.
- Avoid heavy use of alcohol.
- Avoid dependency on drugs.
- Wear seat belts.
- Avoid exposure to known environmental health hazards.
- Take steps to control stress and improve relationships.

It all boils down to this: Live a healthy lifestyle. It's the best way of all to stay out of the hospital.

In my mind no book on how to stay out of the hospital would be complete without a chapter on the best advice of all—staying well. But following only a few of my rules won't do it. You should follow them all. But I'd be willing to wager that you don't. So let's take them one at a time. I'll prove to you how important they are to a sickness-free (and, therefore, hospital-free!) life.

GET PLENTY OF EXERCISE

Exercise improves circulation, lowers blood pressure, improves muscle strength, increases endurance, and improves emotional well-being. There are *many* reasons to exercise regularly. For the present, it can make you look and feel better; for the future, it can reduce your chances of developing many maladies—from osteoporosis to stroke. According to one cardiologist, you double your risk of having a heart attack if you don't get regular exercise.

Actually, as a nation, we seem to be exercising more than ever. Consider the popularity of fitness centers, health spas, cross-country skiing trails, marathons, and triathlon events. But the trouble with these activities is that they cost money and can't always be conveniently done every day. So forget the glamour activities where the outfit is the thing, and forget the super challenges like marathons or triathlons (unless that's your passion in life). There's no need to spend a fortune on sophisticated equipment or fancy spas. The best way to derive the benefits of regular exercise is by some of the simplest and best type of aerobic workouts around—walking, swimming, or bicycling.

DON'T SMOKE

More than 20 years ago, the Surgeon General of the United States Public Health Service announced the conclusion that cigarette smoking was the leading cause of lung cancer. The American Cancer Society has concurred, estimating that cigarette smoking is responsible for 83 percent of lung cancer in men and 43 percent in women—more than 75 percent overall. Smoking has also been implicated in other cancers.

The American Heart Association has stated that smoking is the single most preventable cause of death or illness from coronary heart disease, peripheral arterial disease, chronic obstructive lung disease, and cancer.

Finally, the American Lung Association had this to say: ". . . we want people to take care of their lungs. And cigarette smoking, without a scientific doubt, is the major cause of long-term lung disease."

You've probably seen these statistics again and again. You probably have heard that people who smoke have a ten times greater chance of getting cancer than people who don't. Overall, smoking causes 30 percent of all cancer deaths. But remind yourself of *this* fact: Once you quit smoking, your risks begin to *decrease at once*.

MAINTAIN NORMAL WEIGHT

Being overweight is often more of a cosmetic or social problem than a medical one unless you're 15 to 20 percent over the average weight that's right for your height or body frame. And some 37 million Americans fit into this category. If you're among them, you are more apt to suffer from heart disease, stroke, postoperative complications, and other problems. For those who are 40 percent or more overweight, there is an increased risk of cancer.

If you already suffer from high blood pressure, heart disease, or a number of other ailments, your doctor may advise you to lose some weight.

There are numerous diets and diet plans that one can try, but the most successful, for the long term, are those plans that are nutritionally sound and emphasize low fat and high fiber intake. Forget the fad diets and *any* quick weight loss scheme. These can do you more harm than good.

For the best weight-loss results, make sure you incorporate daily exercise in your program.

FOLLOW A SENSIBLE DIET

Grandma was right: "You are what you eat."

But Americans are so obsessed with diets and dieting, that it's often difficult to know what is and what is not good nutrition.

Let's go back to the basics of nutrition. It's not necessary to memorize the nutrient composition of foods in order to have a nutritionally adequate diet. The basics are simple.

A daily food plan for an adult should include:

- Two servings of milk or milk products
- Two to three servings of meat, poultry, or fish
- Four servings of fruits and vegetables
- Four servings of bread, cereal, or grain.

These minimum servings probably would supply less than 1,500 calories a day. Many people will need more calories than the basic food plan allows—some will need slightly less. To see how you "shape up," keep a food diary for at least a week. Write down *everything* you eat, showing the amounts and time you eat.

If you're counting calories, it's best to increase your activity level rather than decrease foods from the basic food groups. In addition, avoid snacking on "empty calories" (cookies, chips, candy). If you must snack, munch on low-calorie foods such as fruit, raw vegetables, or popcorn—unbuttered, of course.

Remember that no single food can provide all the nutrients your body needs. A diet that is varied is most nutritious. Learn enough about foods to know that ice cream is not as good a substitute for milk as yogurt is (regular ice cream has a high amount of fat and refined sugar, therefore more calories, and its calcium content is about one-half that of milk). A basic nutrition textbook is a wise investment for every family. There are several titles suggested later in this chapter.

AVOID HEAVY USE OF ALCOHOL

Use of alcohol takes a heavy toll. Consider these statistics:

- In the United States, traffic accidents are the major cause of violent death. Between 35 and 64 percent of the drivers in fatal accidents had been drinking prior to the accident. Between 45 and 60 percent of all fatal crashes involving a young driver are alcohol related.
- As many as 50 percent of those who died in falling accidents had been drinking.
- Approximately one-half of adult fire deaths involve alcohol. Alcoholics were found to be ten times more likely to die in fires than the general population.
- Alcohol plays a significant role in drownings. One study reported that 68 percent of drowning victims had been drinking and another study reported that 50 percent of such victims had been drinking.
- Alcoholics are at particularly high risk of committing suicide. Between 15 and 64 percent of suicide attempters and up to 80 percent of suicides had been drinking at the time of the event. The risk of suicide for alcoholics is as much as 30 times greater than the risk of suicide for the general population.

These statistics are very sobering. They are extracted from the Fourth Special Report to the U.S. Congress on Alcohol and Health prepared by the U.S. Department of Health and Human Services, Public Health Service. Additionally, this report points out the medical consequences of alcohol use, and these are also worth examining:

- Long-standing use of substantial amounts of alcohol has been found in a large proportion of patients with unexplained heart muscle disease.

- Brief drinking sprees in apparently healthy individuals can result in premature heartbeats or total loss of rhythmic beating in the heart's upper chambers.
- Epidemiologic studies show that in all races and both sexes, regular consumption of large amounts of alcohol is associated with a substantially higher prevalence of high blood pressure.
- Alcohol use is associated with stroke, phlebitis, and varicose veins, and also may be involved in an unusual form of angina pectoris (chest pain), which is widely believed to be due to spasms in large coronary arteries.
- Numerous studies have shown that both bingeing and long-term imbibing result in lowered testosterone levels in the serum of males. The reduced testosterone level causes sexual impotence, loss of libido, breast enlargement, loss of facial hair, and testicular atrophy in many male alcoholics.
- Brain dysfunction is considered to be one of the major consequences of alcoholism. In any given sample of alcoholics, the proportion of individuals with brain atrophy ranges from 50 percent to 100 percent, depending on the selectivity of the alcoholism treatment program from which the sample is drawn.
- Heavy alcohol consumption has been related to increased risk of cancer at various sites in the human body, especially the mouth, pharynx, larynx, and esophagus. Cancer risk is further increased for heavy drinkers who also use tobacco.
- The positive association between liver cancer and alcohol consumption is related to cirrhosis; very often the cancer is preceded or accompanied by cirrhosis or hepatitis and infection.
- A rapidly growing body of literature provides evidence that abusive drinking during pregnancy is potentially detrimental to the development of the human fetus. Effects may range from mild physical and behavioral deficits to fetal alcohol syndrome (FAS). The major features of FAS are mental retardation, poor motor development, extreme growth deficiency before birth and throughout childhood, and a characteristic cluster of facial abnormalities. Besides the problem of FAS, studies have consistently found that heavier alcohol use during pregnancy is associated with decreased birth weight, greater frequency of spontaneous abortion, and behavioral and neurological effects on newborns.

AVOID DEPENDENCY ON DRUGS

Any drug, taken in excess, can act as a poison in your body. Nevertheless some are obviously more harmful than others. The "hard" drugs and narcotics (such as heroin, cocaine, morphine, and Demerol) have the potential for fatal overdose. Addiction is one of the most serious medical and social problems of our time.

Some of the most abused legal, doctor-prescribed drugs are amphetamines, tranquilizers, and sedatives.

Amphetamines, "speed" or "uppers," stimulate the body and seem to give a person extra energy. Unfortunately, these drugs also increase some forms of heart disease by constricting small blood vessels, and they cause severe mood changes. Because amphetamines are now known to be potentially dangerous, their use is much more tightly controlled and physicians seldom prescribe them. There is no medical use for amphetamines, and they should not be taken as an adjunct to dieting.

Tranquilizers, or "downers," have been the most popularly prescribed mood-changing drugs. Some of the common tranquilizers include diazepam (Valium), chlordiazepoxide hydrochloride (Librium), and meprobamate (Equanil or Miltown). These drugs were frequently prescribed for persons who were nervous or anxious, but they had a band-aid effect (at best) for the underlying problems and often created new problems that were very serious. These have been widely publicized. Tranquilizers are still prescribed, and patients can become dependent on them. Also, because one tablet of Valium or Librium has the sedative effect of one alcoholic drink, driving a car while taking the medicine can be unsafe, and drinking alcohol while taking these tranquilizers can be deadly.

Major tranquilizers are used for serious emotional disturbances and may have a depressant effect on the central nervous system. According to the FDA, these tranquilizers, taken with alcohol, can cause additional depression to central nervous system functions, which, in turn, can result in severe impairment of walking or using the hands. The combination also can produce severe and possibly fatal depression of the respiratory system. Heavy drinking in combination with the major tranquilizers may increase the potential for liver damage.

Sedatives/hypnotics are another group of drugs that should not be prescribed or taken as often as they are. Sedatives seldom produce a restful sleep, and the next morning's hangover can be very uncomfortable. Sedatives are habit forming, and an overdose can kill. A report of the National Institute of Alcohol Abuse and Alcoholism cites a study which found that the lethal dose of barbiturates was nearly 50 percent lower when taken with alcohol than when taken alone. Other prescription drugs, such as painkillers, can by themselves cause difficulty driving, and taken with alcohol, can cause serious disturbances.

The list can go on. In fact, of the 100 most frequently prescribed drugs, over half contain at least one ingredient known to react adversely with alcohol. Many over-the-counter drugs have the same effect. Information from the Drug Abuse Warning Network (DAWN) shows that more than 47,000 people who have taken alcohol in combination with other drugs are treated in hospital emergency rooms every year. More than 2,500 deaths annually are attributed to alcohol-drug combinations.

These facts are not meant to throw the average person into a panic. There are many occasions when drugs *need* to be taken to make you feel better or even save your life. I hope, however, that the preceding information will make you aware that there can be devastating reactions from drugs.

What's your recourse? Before taking a prescribed drug, ask your physician what the drug is expected to do and what its side effects are. What will happen if you *don't* take it? Is there a less risky drug that may be tried first? If you do decide to take the medicine, what foods or beverages should you avoid?

Take your medication as prescribed by the doctor. If you have a tendency to forget things, write out your medication schedule and tape it to your refrigerator. When a drug label reads "take as needed," it doesn't mean as frequently as you want. Ask the physician (or pharmacist) what is the maximum amount that can safely be taken in one day. When taking prescription drugs, don't take any additional over-the-counter medication without consulting your physician.

When taking medication, you should contact your physician if you experience any of the following side effects: nausea, vomiting, diarrhea, loss of appetite, skin rash, sore throat, dizziness, shortness of breath, faintness or weakness (this list is not meant to be inclusive—if *any* untoward reactions occur, you should seek medical care).

Finally, read the labels on over-the-counter remedies and the package inserts that come with prescription drugs. Buy a *Physicians'*

Desk Reference or other drug book (see "Health Books No Home Should Be Without" on pages 206–7) and study up on the drugs that have been prescribed for you. Take only those drugs that are needed. Remember that the ultimate responsibility for what you put inside your body is *yours*.

WEAR SEAT BELTS

On September 11, 1984, country-western singer Barbara Mandrell and her two children, ages 8 and 14, were in an automobile accident in Hendersonville, Tennessee (near Nashville). Mandrell's Jaguar was hit head-on by another car whose driver was killed. Moments before the crash Mandrell and her children had buckled their seat belts, and this preventive measure is credited with saving their lives.

According to the National Safety Council, one out of four auto deaths is caused by ejection and could be totally prevented if drivers and passengers used seat belts. In front-end crashes (as Mandrell experienced) or roll-over accidents, seat belts also reduce the amount of injury that occurs. (Mandrell's leg was broken and her knee badly cut; her children were unharmed.) Becoming paralyzed, losing the sight of an eye, suffering severe head injuries—these are often the penalties that people pay when they don't use lap and shoulder belts.

Ask a paramedic or a policeman or an emergency room worker about it. They're the ones who pick up the pieces after an automobile accident. They'll tell you: Buckle up!

AVOID EXPOSURE TO KNOWN ENVIRONMENTAL HEALTH HAZARDS

For many years safe drinking water and clean air were taken for granted in this country. No more. As our country has become more urbanized and industrialized, we have polluted the water we drink and the air we breathe. Everyone's health is affected by these modern-day problems, but again, some people are more at risk than others.

In recent years some household water supplies have been contaminated with herbicides, pesticides, acids, and other pollutants. How can you be sure that the water *you're* drinking is safe?

It's not always a simple matter to find the answer to that question. You could call your municipal water supply office and find out what's in the drinking water. However, that might not help much, since many municipalities don't do a detailed analysis and may not have the information you want.

If you're really concerned about the purity of your drinking supply, it would probably be easiest to take a sample of the water yourself and send it to a private laboratory for analysis. Then you could compare the laboratory results with the federal regulations for safe limits. How do you find these safe-limit numbers? By contacting your regional water management office. If you don't know how to get in touch with that office, you can contact the Environmental Protection Agency (EPA) for the number (call toll-free: 1-800-424-9065).

If the safety of your supply of drinking water is in doubt, you should drink and cook with bottled water until the problem is corrected.

As elusive as contaminated water is to detect, it's pretty easy to tell when the air you're breathing is not up to par. For a person with an existing lung problem, breathing polluted air can be devastating. Air pollution contributes to the cause of certain lung conditions (lung cancer and emphysema), and once the disease is established, pollution makes the problems worse. Any person concerned about his or her health should not live in a heavily industrialized area or an area that has a significant number of days when pollution reaches dangerous levels.

Other public health hazards that you should be aware of:

Avoid working around chemical and radiation hazards without adequate protection. Avoid unnecessary exposure to x-rays and other radiation sources. Avoid too much sunlight (wear protective clothing, use a sunscreen). Safety-proof your home against falls and accidents, fires, and poisonings. Avoid drowning by learning and following water safety rules. Avoid food-borne illness by following safe practices in food preparation and serving.

TAKE STEPS TO CONTROL STRESS AND IMPROVE RELATIONSHIPS

You're late for a business appointment and the traffic seems to be moving at a snail's pace. The knucklehead in front of you is going 40 mph in a 50 mph zone. You tailgate for a while, hoping he will move faster, but he doesn't get the message. You tap on the steering wheel and mutter a few unkind words. Finally you gun the engine and whip around the guy, narrowly missing the car coming in the other direction. You wipe the sweat off your brow, then glance at your watch. Already five minutes late and five more miles to go.

As you push on, your head is racing with thoughts of getting there, presenting the material, getting the account. Then your mind goes back to the office and the boss. Who does he think he is, anyway? Today's memo, for example: "A reminder: You're not paid to think!" Just remembering it, you clench your teeth and feel that gnawing pain in your stomach. You probably should have eaten lunch but there'll be time for a candy bar after the appointment. Those days of leisurely lunches are long gone.

Recognize anyone in this slice of life? Do you find yourself working under pressure, never having time to enjoy life, frequently feeling hostile and out of sorts? Then what you're probably suffering from is stress.

Stress is that collection of "fight or flight" responses—increased heart rate and blood pressure, rapid breathing and increased muscle tension—that would seem most appropriate if a lion were chasing you. But is it appropriate to act this way when you read the boss's nasty memo (and you need the job) or when you're frustrated by slow traffic (and you're late for an appointment)?

Stress is one of the dilemmas of 20th-century man and it can cause significant health problems or make existing conditions worse. Stress is a suspected ingredient in migraine headache, backache, insomnia, high blood pressure, ulcer, asthma attacks, heart disease, and cancer. But is it really the stress that causes the troubles or your reaction to it?

You *can* defeat the stress monster by changing your perception of events and how you react to them. Suppose, for example, you're a working woman who's also the mother of two boys, aged six and eight. It's a busy Tuesday morning at work and you get a call from the school nurse. Six-year-old Johnny has a temperature of 102 degrees and his cold is much worse. "Could you please come to school and pick up Johnny?"

You stare at the mountain of work and wonder why today, of all days, Johnny has to be sick. It's just not fair. You kick the trash can and stuff papers in a briefcase.

Once home with Johnny, though, you realize how nice it is to be with this second child who doesn't always get enough of your time and attention. You read to Johnny, listen to his stories about school and soccer. While he's napping, you even get some work done.

If you had focused on the fact that you missed a day of work, that would be stressful. But the focus is now on the nonstressful rewarding day that you spent with your son. Many bad (stressful) events can be turned around this way.

Here are some other tips to defuse stress:

Live Healthy—Eating regular, well-balanced meals, not smoking, getting regular exercise—these can help with stress reduction.

Get Adequate Sleep—Without sufficient sleep, it's difficult to handle the stresses of life. The late movie on TV isn't worth the next day's fatigue.

Relax during the Day—To reduce stress, you can practice deep breathing exercises, Transcendental Meditation, yoga, biofeedback, or behavior modification. These relaxation techniques have helped many people, but they may require professional assistance or classroom time to learn the skills. Most of us have favorite activities that help us to relax, such as getting a massage, taking a catnap, or going to a movie or out to dinner. Take time to do those things. Indulge yourself a little and enjoy some of the pleasures of life. There'll never be a better time than *now*.

Talk It Over—If you have a trusted friend you can talk things over with, you're indeed fortunate. The stressors, the problems of life, are always easier when you can unburden them to someone who understands. It's unfortunate that so many people today have to rely on professional counselors and therapists to talk over their troubles. In many cases, all a person needs is a sympathetic friend.

TYPES OF PREVENTION

The preceding nine health tips all fall into the category of *primary prevention*. This is the least costly and most effective form of prevention, and as you may notice, these principles can be followed without assistance from the medical establishment. Primary prevention is the ideal—disease is prevented by modifying certain risk factors or altering a person's resistance to disease. But primary prevention is very difficult to accomplish because the benefits of good health practices are not always seen immediately.

Secondary prevention is early intervention or detecting sickness in its earliest stages. If your local hospital or service organization sponsors a health fair and you take advantage of the event, you might find that your blood pressure is elevated, or if you're a woman, that your Pap test shows atypical cells. Before you went to the health fair, you had no symptoms that would suggest high blood pressure or localized cancer of the cervix. But, fortunately, since you now know you have a problem, you can get treatment while the disease is in its early stages and your chances of a cure are much improved. This is an example of secondary prevention.

Tertiary prevention is the most expensive and the least effective form of prevention. It is the stage when the medical establishment is most likely to be involved. Tertiary prevention is the treatment of an established disease to prevent relapse or further deterioration. Treatment for lung cancer, for example, is expensive, painful, and not always effective. Yet lung cancer must be treated to prevent spread, or metastasis, to other parts of the body. So the surgery and other therapy may be considered tertiary prevention.

It's a known fact that American physicians and hospitals get the most money not if they keep people healthy, but if they treat patients in the most expensive possible way after they have become ill. I say this not to suggest that all doctors and hospitals are greedy—most are not. The problem lies not with the individual physician, but at the very roots of medical philosophy and education. Medical students receive almost no instruction in preventive medicine.

RISKS AND
TESTS FOR DIFFERENT AGES

What are the major risks to your health and what can you do about them?

Each age and stage in a person's life has its problems and priorities and each age has certain health risk factors that are more important than others. Here's what to look out for in the different stages of your adult life.

Prevention Starts in Your 20s

These are the risk-taking years when driving fast and drinking too much can cause immediate problems and when the bad habits of smoking, indiscriminate sex, and poor nutrition can cause problems later on. The 20s may be the last opportunity to easily change health habits *for the better,* so these may be considered the most important years if a person wants to make it to a healthy old age.

Unless there are known health problems, there is no reason for a regular physical examination during this decade. Yearly physicals, in fact, are seldom warranted until the 50s. What *is* needed, though, are regular selective screening tests, and many of these can be obtained at free clinics or health fairs.

In this country, 35 million people suffer from hypertension or high blood pressure. It can be a silent killer. Beginning in the 20s, every person should have the blood pressure checked every two years. Normal blood pressure is 120/80. High blood pressure is considered 160/90 or higher. The higher the blood pressure, the greater the risk of heart disease, stroke, and kidney disease.

If you do have high blood pressure (at any age), you should be under the care of a physician. He may first recommend changes in diet (reduce calories, cholesterol, and salt) and an exercise program. If these measures don't bring down the blood pressure, then drugs may be prescribed to lower it.

Beginning in the late teens or at age 20, every women should have two consecutive yearly Pap tests, and if these are negative, the test can be dropped to once every three years. This recommendation comes from the American Cancer Society.

Also from the Cancer Society is the recommendation that a physician should perform a breast examination every three years from age 20 to age 40 and every year after age 40. Beginning in the 20s it's a good health practice for every woman to examine her breasts once a month about a week after the menstrual period. The risk of breast cancer is not very high in the 20s (the 50s are the high-risk years), but breast self-examination is a good habit to acquire. If you're uncertain how to examine your breasts, you can learn the proper method from your nurse or doctor or through literature from the American Cancer Society or classes conducted by the Cancer Society and other nonprofit organizations. Breast diagnostic centers (also called breast care centers) help women—for a fee—to learn proper self-examination techniques. This is part of an overall program to encourage early diagnosis for the most effective treatment of breast problems. Women who have attended these intensive sessions have found them very worthwhile.

Physicians at New Jersey's Hunterdon Medical Center advise doing a blood cholesterol test every four years beginning in the 20s until age 60 and none thereafter. High cholesterol levels increase the likelihood of heart attack. According to the American Heart Association, cholesterol levels should be 180 for persons under 25, 200 for persons 25 to 45, and 220 for those over 45 years old. Cholesterol levels can be reduced by modifying the diet and cutting down on foods that are high in cholesterol and animal fat.

The 30s—The Responsible Years

In this decade, the risk-taking side of life becomes less important as a career and family responsibilities take top priority. This decade is a time when proper diet and regular exercise must be "sandwiched in." Women need to make a conscious effort to get more calcium in their diet to prevent debilitating osteoporosis later in life, and men need to avoid heavy fatty diets that raise cholesterol levels and narrow arteries.

Some doctors recommend a first base-line mammogram for women between the ages of 35 and 40, at the time of the regular gynecological examination. (A mammogram is a low-dose breast x-ray that can find cancers too small to be felt by hand.)

The 40s—Midlife Problems

For some, this may seem like the beginning of the end. Some may be plagued with backaches, especially if they're overweight and don't exercise. Heart attacks for men begin in this decade. Women may get breast cancer, and both men and women are susceptible to cancer of the rectum and lung cancer. The 40s is the time of the "midlife crisis."

Beginning in the 40s, every man and woman should have the stool examined annually for blood. Bowel cancers usually cause slight bleeding, which produces a color change when a speck of stool is placed on a treated paper card. This test can pick up early colon cancer. As of December 1984, home testing kits for signs of bowel and rectal cancer could be purchased at drugstores, and the test can be done at home.

Also in the 40s a tonometry, or test for glaucoma, should be done every three to five years. This regular testing should continue indefinitely. Glaucoma causes pressure within the eye, which leads to constriction of vision and even blindness. If, during examination, your eye tension is elevated, then you should be under the care of an ophthalmologist (eye doctor) who can prescribe proper treatment (usually in the form of eye drops).

Lifestyle Catches Up in the 50s

These ten years intensify the problems of the 40s with more cases of heart attack and cancer taking their toll. For men, this is the time for coronary bypass surgery or coronary care units. Lung cancer and emphysema result from years of smoking. Alcohol abuse brings on cirrhosis of the liver. In the 50s there's increased risk of prostate cancer for men, breast and cervical cancer for women, and bowel cancer for both sexes. For these reasons, annual physical examinations begin to make more sense, so that diseases can be discovered and treated early.

60s and Beyond—When Life Can Be Kind

If you've maintained a healthy lifestyle and have friends and interests that keep you active and involved, this can be one of the best decades of your life.

If you are fortunate to reach these "golden years" in relatively good health, you might give some of the credit to "good genes" or a healthy ancestry. Heredity is certainly a factor in longevity and quality of life.

As a person passes the seventh decade, there is increased incidence of chronic disease and the constant threat of cancer. This means that health supervision and medical care assume a greater priority in life.

The importance of quality health care for the elderly cannot be underestimated. In 1982 in the United States, the life expectancy was 78.2 years for women and 70.8 years for men. Our population is definitely getting grayer.

Some physicians recommend regular tests for blood glucose (sugar), complete blood count (which includes hemoglobin and hematocrit levels), blood urea nitrogen (a test to detect kidney disease), and other blood tests—besides cholesterol levels—for determining risk of heart disease. In addition, some recommend systematic skin testing for tuberculosis, regular electrocardiograms, urinalysis, and proctosigmoidoscopy (examination of the lower intestinal tract). Fewer recommend routine chest x-rays. As regular screening procedures, these are all subject to debate. The tests I've already mentioned and the time interval between tests are generally accepted as being most important and most cost effective.

CARING FOR YOUR OWN MINOR AILMENTS

If everyone who had a headache or cold sought medical attention, there wouldn't be enough doctors available to see them. Furthermore, there's seldom a need to seek a physician's advice when the flu or a minor stomach ache occurs. That's because these maladies cannot be "cured" but must run their course. They are "self-limited" illnesses that will go away by themselves. The vast majority of patients who physicians see suffer from self-limited disease. Many patients, of course, want the emotional assurance of knowing that they just have a cold rather than pneumonia, or a stomach ache rather than a bleeding ulcer, and if they want to pay for this self-indulgence, I guess that's their privilege. However, needless visits to the doctor are expensive in time and money, and sometimes such visits persuade doctors to prescribe tests or medications that aren't necessary.

To avoid unnecessary trips to the doctor, every person needs to act, to a certain extent, as his or her own diagnostician. A good rule of thumb: If symptoms persist or become worse, it's a good idea to see a physician. Also, you might want to invest in a few reputable self-care health books. Using the information in these as a base line, you can determine if your problem is more serious. If it is, you should seek medical attention. If you have a chronic illness that is affected by common ailments, ask your physician what guidelines you should following regarding visits.

HEALTH BOOKS NO HOME SHOULD BE WITHOUT

Child Care

Brazelton, T. Berry. *Infants and Mothers: Differences in Development.* New York: Dell Publishing Co., 1983.

———. *Toddlers and Parents: A Declaration of Independence.* New York: Dell Publishing Co., 1976.

Green, Martin I. *A Sigh of Relief: The Revised Edition of the First Aid Handbook for Childhood Emergencies.* New York: Bantam Books, 1984.

Spock, Benjamin. *Baby and Child Care.* New York: Pocket Books, 1976.

First Aid

American Medical Association. *The AMA Handbook of First Aid and Emergency Care.* New York: Random House, 1980.

General Health Care

Kunz, Jeffrey R. M., ed. *The American Medical Association Family Medical Guide.* New York: Random House, 1982.

Vickery, Donald, and James Fries. *Take Care of Yourself: A Consumer's Guide to Medical Care.* Reading, Mass.: Addison-Wesley Publishing Co., 1981.

Nutrition

Brody, Jane. *Jane Brody's Nutrition Book.* New York: Bantam Books, 1982.

Kruetler, Patricia. *Nutrition in Perspective.* Englewood Cliffs, N.J.: Prentice-Hall, 1980.

Reference

American Pharmaceutical Association. *Handbook of Nonprescription Drugs.* American Pharmaceutical Association, 1982.

Berkow, Robert, ed. *The Merck Manual.* 14th ed. Rahway, N.J.: Merck, 1982.

Dorland's Illustrated Medical Dictionary. 26th ed. Philadelphia: W. B. Saunders Co., 1981.

Gennaro, Alphonso R., ed. *Blakiston's Pocket Medical Dictionary.* 4th ed. New York: McGraw-Hill, 1979.

Goss, Charles M., ed. *Gray's Anatomy of the Human Body.* 29th ed. Philadelphia: Lea & Febiger, 1973.

Physicians' Desk Reference. 39th ed. Oradell, N.J.: Medical Economics Books, 1985.

Thomas, Clayton L. *Taber's Cyclopedic Medical Dictionary.* 14th ed. Philadelphia: F. A. Davis Co., 1981.

INDEX

Rodale Press, Inc., publishes PREVENTION®, the better health magazine.
For information on how to order your subscription,
write to PREVENTION®, Emmaus, PA 18049.